Inside the
2009
Influenza
Pandemic

Inside the 2009 Influenza Pandemic

Jon Stuart Abramson

Wake Forest University School of Medicine, USA

World Scientific

NEW JERSEY · LONDON · SINGAPORE · BEIJING · SHANGHAI · HONG KONG · TAIPEI · CHENNAI

Published by

World Scientific Publishing Co. Pte. Ltd.

5 Toh Tuck Link, Singapore 596224

USA office: 27 Warren Street, Suite 401-402, Hackensack, NJ 07601

UK office: 57 Shelton Street, Covent Garden, London WC2H 9HE

Library of Congress Cataloging-in-Publication Data
Abramson, Jon Stuart.
    Inside the 2009 influenza pandemic / Jon Stuart Abramson.
        p. ; cm.
    Inside the two thousand nine influenza pandemic
    Includes bibliographical references and index.
    ISBN-13: 978-981-4324-10-6 (hardcover : alk. paper)
    ISBN-10: 981-4324-10-8 (hardcover : alk. paper)
    1. Influenza--Epidemiology. 2. Influenza--Prevention. 3. Emergency management.
I. Title. II. Title: Inside the two thousand nine influenza pandemic.
    [DNLM: 1. Influenza, Human--epidemiology. 2. Influenza, Human--prevention& control.
3. Communicable Disease Control--organization & administration. 4. Disaster Planning--
organization & administration. 5. Disease Outbreaks--prevention & control. 6. Influenza A Virus,
H1N1 Subtype. WC 515]
    RA644.I6A27 2010
    614.5'18--dc22
                                                                          2010043492

British Library Cataloguing-in-Publication Data
A catalogue record for this book is available from the British Library.

Typeset by Stallion Press
Email: enquiries@stallionpress.com

Printed in Singapore.

Dedication

To my wife Cynthia who affords me the time to pursue my various academic interests and my children Melissa, Rebecca and Seth whose presence reminds me each day why children are the foundation of our aspirations. To my many colleagues who share the vision that prevention of disease, rather than cure, is the ultimate goal.

Contents

Abbreviations

2009 H1N1 virus — The quadruple reassortant influenza A (H1N1) virus that caused the 2009 pandemic

ACIP — Advisory Committee on Immunization Practices of the Centers for Disease Control and Prevention

ARDS — Acute Respiratory Distress Syndrome

BMI — Body mass index

CDC — Centers for Disease Control and Prevention (United States of America)

ECMO — Extracorporeal membrane oxygenation

GBS — Guillain–Barré syndrome

HA — Hemagglutinin protein

HCW — Healthcare worker

ICU — Intensive care unit

LAIV — Live attenuated influenza vaccine

NA — Neuraminidase protein

PICU — Pediatric intensive care unit

RT-PCR — Reverse transcription-polymerase chain reaction

SAGE — Strategic Advisory Group of Experts on Immunization to the World Health Organization

SARS — Severe Acute Respiratory Syndrome

The Strategy — The US National Strategy for Pandemic Influenza

TIV — Trivalent inactivated influenza virus vaccine

WHO — World Health Organization

Prologue

I hung up the phone and chills shot up my spine. Although I knew the call would someday come, the immediate surge of emotions was surprisingly very strong. There was little doubt that Dr. Chris Ohl, an adult infectious disease specialist who was on the other end of the line, also understood the potential impact of the information he was conveying and the emotion in his voice was telling. He had just been informed at a meeting of the North Carolina and South Carolina Health Departments that a new reassortant influenza virus containing genetic material from birds, pigs and humans (designated the 2009 H1N1 virus in this book) had been rapidly spreading and causing disease in large numbers of people in Mexico since March 2009. And now, a month later, the virus had crossed the border into the United States of America.

For the past three decades, I have been on the faculty at Wake Forest University School of Medicine as a pediatric infectious disease specialist. My job encompasses clinical care, teaching, research and administration with the majority of my research time focused in the area of influenza. During the past 15 years I had been Chair of the American Academy of Pediatrics Committee on Infectious Diseases, then Chair of the Centers for Disease Control and Prevention (CDC) Advisory Committee on Immunization Practices (ACIP), and I currently serve on the World Health Organization (WHO) Strategic Advisory Group of Experts on Immunization (SAGE), including the Ad Hoc Policy Advisory SAGE Working Group on Influenza A (H1N1) Vaccines. During this time I have participated in many meetings about pandemic influenza planning, including meetings where we were asked to advise the US Secretary of Health and

Human Services and the WHO Director-General on how to prioritize the use of influenza vaccines once a pandemic had begun. All this background information is meant only to say that I knew enough to be concerned that this 2009 H1N1 virus could cause the next pandemic and if this occurred all of the pandemic plans would soon be tested. What I did not know was whether at the end of this pandemic we would have passed or failed this test.

Chapter 1

Epidemic and Pandemic Influenza: Background Information

"The virus writes the rules and this one, like all influenza viruses, can change the rules, without rhyme or reason, at any time."

Dr. Margaret Chan, Director-General of the
World Health Organization, announcing the
start of the 2009 influenza pandemic, June 11, 2009

1.1 Background Information on Influenza Epidemics and Pandemics

A KEY POINT: Influenza viruses mutate frequently and on occasion the genes will mutate or reassort in a way that produces a very potent warrior capable of infecting most of the world's population.

1.1.1 *Influenza Viruses*

Influenza viruses are named by a standard nomenclature that specifies the virus type (A, B or C), geographical location where first isolated, sequential number of isolation, year of isolation and hemagglutinin (HA) and neuraminidase (NA) protein subtypes. For example, the strain that has been used to make the monovalent 2009 pandemic vaccine is designated A/California/7/2009 (H1N1) which indicates that it is an influenza A

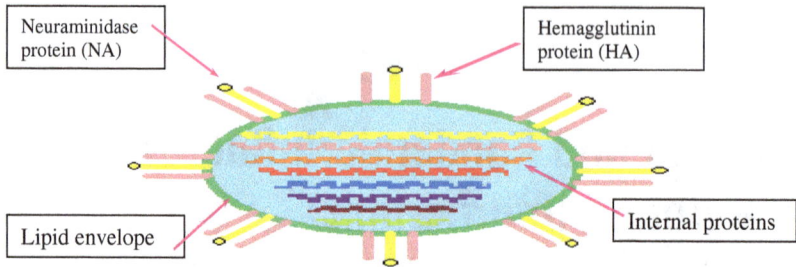

Fig. 1. Influenza viral structure. The HA and NA are genetically unstable proteins on the outside of the influenza virus lipid envelope and these proteins can undergo frequent changes. The internal proteins (polymerase PB2, polymerase PB1, polymerase PA, nuclear protein, matrix proteins and nonstructural protein) do not undergo frequent changes.

virus, isolated in California, the seventh strain so isolated in 2009 and is an H1N1 subtype.

The structure of the influenza virus is composed of eight genetically stable proteins contained internally, a transmembrane protein and two proteins attached to the outside of the membrane that are subject to a high rate of genetic mutation during viral replication (Fig. 1). The internal proteins serve a number of functions including determining whether a particular virus is an A, B or C influenza virus. Influenza A and B are common causes of human disease and influenza A typically causes the more severe disease. Influenza C only rarely causes disease in humans.

The hemagglutinin (HA) and neuraminidase (NA) are the two external proteins. The HA protein allows attachment and membrane fusion of the virus with host cells. When the HA undergoes a genetic mutation or recombination (e.g., HA genes from two or more viruses recombine to yield an altered HA protein) the HA structure can change and thereby avoid an antibody immune response without affecting its ability to bind to the receptor. The NA protein can also undergo genetic mutation or recombination. The NA digests sialic acid which most cells have on their surface. The removal of sialic acid from the host receptor enables the virus to gain entry into the host cell. The virus then reproduces in the host cell and the NA removal of sialic acid also helps the virus progeny be released from the cell.

Humoral IgG and mucosal IgA antibodies are important in protecting against influenza. Neutralizing antibody to the HA protein is most important since this antibody can block the attachment of the virus to host cells and thereby prevent disease from occurring. However, if a person has not been infected with a particular subtype of influenza virus (e.g., H1N1) before or has been infected with this subtype, but the HA has undergone a significant genetic-induced structural change, then the person is at risk for infection. Antibody to the NA protein is also thought to offer some protection by delaying the spread of the virus to other cells. IgG antibodies persist longer than IgA antibodies and play a more important role in long-term immunity.[1]

There are 16 HA and 9 NA proteins and each of these have been found in at least one animal species, but only some HA and NA types cause widespread human transmission (Table 1).

Table 1. The HA and NA Proteins Present in Influenza Virus Subtypes are Noted As Well As Whether They Cause Infection Only in Animals or Also in Humans

HA subtype	Human	Animal	NA subtype	Human	Animal
1	+	+	1	+	+
2	+	+	2	+	+
3	+	+	3		+
4		+	4		+
5	+	+	5		+
6		+	6		+
7	+	+	7	+	+
8		+	8		+
9	+	+	9		+
10		+			
11		+			
12		+			
13		+			
14		+			
15		+			
16		+			

The various HA and NA proteins that have been found to occur in nature could potentially result in the emergence of 144 (16 x 9) different influenza virus HA and NA combinations. However, only six types of HA proteins and three types of NA proteins have been found to cause influenza A disease in humans and the vast majority of disease has been due to influenza viruses with H1N1, H2N2 or H3N2 subtypes. For the most part the reason why people are infected with influenza viruses multiple times during their lifetime relates to changes that occur in the genetically unstable external proteins.

The terms "antigenic drift" and "antigenic shift" are used to describe the extent of the genetic changes that occur to the HA and NA proteins. Antigenic drift is due to point mutations that accumulate over time. These point mutations can lead to structural changes in the HA or NA that cause an individual who was previously immune to the original strain not to be immune to the drifted protein because the antibodies created as part of the immune response to the previous influenza virus infection do not neutralize the external proteins of the mutated virus. Antigenic drift results in sporadic outbreaks and limited epidemics because the majority of the population has pre-existing antibodies that still provide at least partial immune protection against the virus. In a typical influenza season the strains have undergone drift, but have not shifted, and a minority of the population is infected with the virus in any given year.

In contrast, antigenic shift is due to reassortment of virus genetic material of two or more influenza virus subtypes. This reassortment can occur between two or more different human influenza virus strains or can be a recombination of genetic material from different species (e.g., the 2009 pandemic virus was a quadravalent reassortant virus that contained genetic material from birds, pigs and humans). Even though the subtype may be the same as in previous influenza seasons, the genetic makeup of the HA or NA of the virus is very different from what is found in the original strain (e.g., the HA protein on the H1N1 seasonal virus that had circulated in recent years was very different from the HA on the 2009 H1N1 pandemic virus and antibodies to this seasonal virus provided no protection against the 2009 pandemic virus). Antigenic shifts cause more widespread epidemics

Table 2. Differences Between Influenza Viruses that Cause Seasonal versus Pandemic Influenza

Seasonal Influenza

— Genetic point mutations lead to small variations in the HA or NA protein structure
— HA and NA proteins are closely related to HA and NA strains from prior years
— A minority (5–15%) of the population is infected with the virus
— Infection rates are variable, but hospitalizations and deaths are increased compared to other times of the year and mostly occur in the elderly and those with underlying chronic diseases

Pandemic Influenza

— Recombinant genetic changes lead to substantial structural changes in the HA or NA proteins
— HA or NA proteins are distinctly different from previous years
— A large percentage (20–50%) the population is infected with the virus
— High infection rates in most, or all, age groups with increased hospitalizations and deaths compared to seasonal influenza

and pandemics, because a greater percentage of the population does not have immunity against this shifted virus (Table 2).

The 2009 pandemic influenza virus, designated in this book by the term "2009 H1N1 virus," is a quadruple reassortant virus containing genetic material from birds, pigs and humans. Pigs are known to act as a mixing vessel where strains of influenza virus from birds, pigs and humans can exchange and reassort genes and create a new virus that has genes that produce internal and external proteins from these species (Figs. 2 and 3). Up until the emergence of the 2009 H1N1 strain in humans, this virus had been circulating in pigs for over a decade, but this strain had not undergone a genetic change that would enable it to spread easily to or between humans. The 2009 H1N1 strain differs from the other double, triple or quadruple reassortant viruses in that this new strain efficiently spreads between humans. It is this ability to easily pass from human to human that enabled this virus to cause the current pandemic. The specific genetic factors that enable a given influenza virus to be easily transmitted among persons are not well understood. The 2009 H1N1 virus does not easily spread between pigs or from pigs to humans, but does seem to spread

5

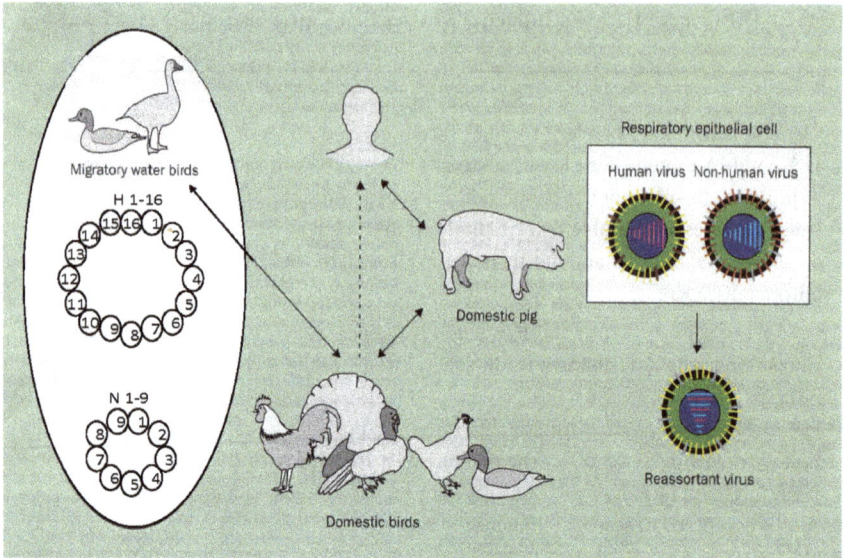

Fig. 2. This diagram depicts how influenza viruses from various species can recombine to form a new virus. The figure was modified from a slide that was previously on the CDC influenza website (www.cdc.gov). Human and bird influenza viruses can infect a pig which acts as the mixing vessel and allows these viruses to recombine to create a new virus that had genetic material from both the bird and human viral strains. In the case of the 2009 pandemic, genetic material from a pig virus, in addition to an avian and human virus, recombined to create the 2009 H1N1 virus.

more readily from humans to pigs. Insufficient historical and geographical data about influenza viruses in swine populations limits the ability to make conclusions about where and when this virus emerged.[2,3]

The 2009 H1N1 virus differs substantially from the avian H5N1 virus that has been circulating amongst the bird population for over a decade and has caused concern that it might cause a pandemic. The avian H5N1 virus has bird and human but no swine genetic material. From 2003 to 2009 there have been <500 confirmed human cases of H5N1 infection in 15 countries in Asia and the Middle East. The great majority of these cases occurred in people who had direct contact with chickens in farms or outdoor poultry markets. The H5N1 virus is highly virulent, with a ~60% mortality, but unlike the 2009 H1N1 virus, has not to date developed the capacity

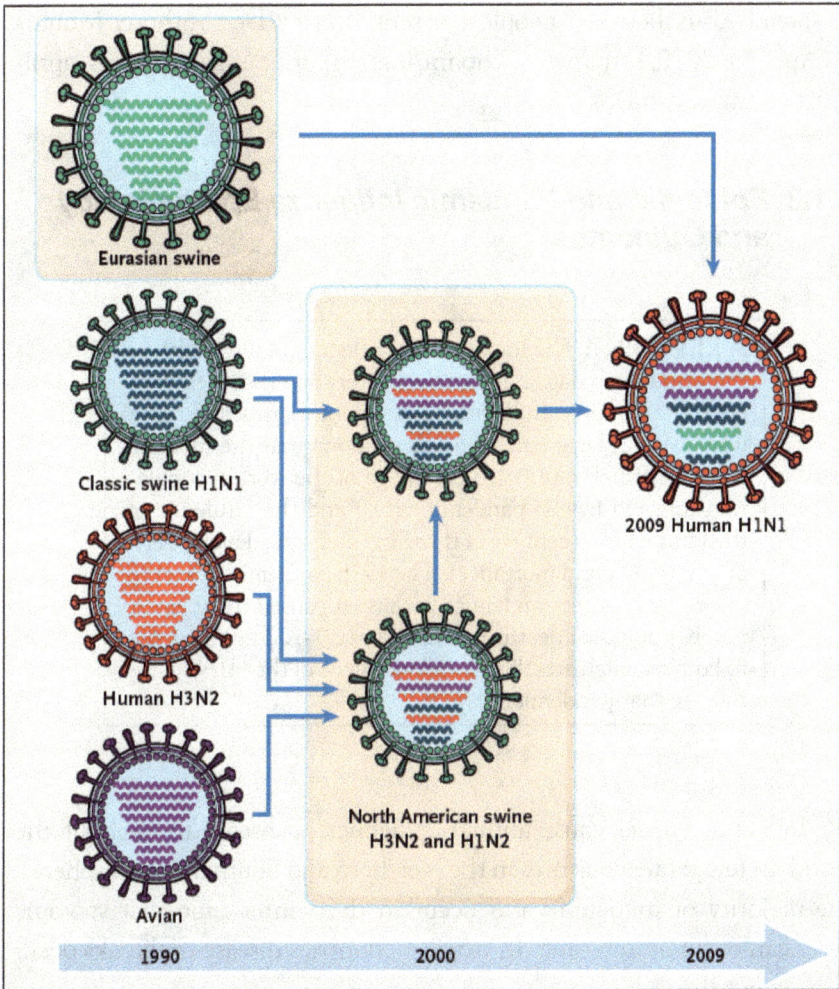

Fig. 3. The history of reassortment events in the evolution of the 2009 H1N1 virus. The eight segments shown within each virus code for the following proteins of the influenza A virus: HA, NA, polymerase PB2, polymerase PB1, polymerase PA, nuclear, matrix and nonstructural proteins. The segments of the human 2009 influenza A (H1N1) virus have coexisted in swine influenza A virus strains for more than 10 years. The ancestors of NA have not been observed for almost 20 years. The mixing vessel for the current reassortment is likely to be a swine host but remains unknown.[4]

to spread easily between people (presentation by Dr. Anthony Mounts on April 14, 2010, http://www.who.int/immunization/sage/ previous_april-2010/en/index.html).

1.1.2 *Epidemic and Pandemic Influenza Epidemiology and Outcomes*

> A KEY POINT: The impact of a pandemic on the health of the world's population is usually greater than that seen with epidemic seasonal influenza. The extent of this difference in impact, in large part, depends on how great the increase is in the attack rate (the percentage of the world's population infected by the pandemic virus) and the virulence of the virus (the percentage of those infected who develop serious morbidity and mortality). The 1918 pandemic was more severe than other pandemics because it caused the greatest number of global deaths (estimated at 50–100 million) due to both the high attack rate and virulence of the H1N1 virus causing that pandemic.

Influenza viruses cause annual epidemics of disease throughout the world. In temperate countries in the Northern and Southern Hemispheres, the majority of influenza cases occur in the winter time, but sporadic cases can occur at any time. In tropical countries disease outbreaks occur throughout the year.

Influenza viruses cause more deaths per year than any other infectious disease in developed countries.[5] In the USA, an average of ∼36,000 influenza-related deaths occur annually (range 17,000–51,000) and this equates to ∼1 out of every 8,300 Americans dying each year due to influenza and its complications. This death toll is greater than that from all other vaccine-preventable diseases combined. While >90% of seasonal influenza-associated deaths occur in the elderly, substantial numbers of children die from influenza and its complications. Chronic diseases that can increase the risk for severe morbidity or mortality due to influenza in children and adults include chronic pulmonary diseases such as asthma and cystic fibrosis, congenital or acquired immunodeficiencies, cancer and other diseases that require immunosuppressive therapy, sickle cell anemia and other hemoglobinopathies, metabolic diseases including diabetes mellitus and renal, liver and hepatic diseases. Some of these children and adolescents have no underlying chronic condition and many of those who die have not been vaccinated against influenza.

Influenza causes an average of ~226,000 hospitalizations in the USA each year (range 55,000–431,000). Influenza H3N2 strains are usually more virulent than H1N1 strains and therefore the higher end of this hospitalization range usually occurs in years where an H3N2 strain predominates. Those >65 years of age account for ~60% of the annual hospitalizations caused by influenza virus. Approximately 20,000 children <5 years of age are hospitalized with those <2 years of age having the highest rates of hospitalization of all age groups. The rate of hospitalization is greater in those with underlying high-risk chronic conditions, but a substantial percentage of children and adults who are hospitalized do not have underlying chronic illnesses. Higher rates of chronic illness in minority populations result in an increased rate of severe disease due to influenza.[5]

In many developing countries, particularly those in tropical parts of the world, the burden of disease has not been well documented, but the studies that have been done suggest that influenza causes greater morbidity and mortality in children and adults than in developed countries.[6] An influenza H3N2 outbreak in Madagascar in July–August of 2001 had a 67% attack rate with ~27,000 cases and 800 deaths with 55% of the deaths being in children <5 years of age. Similarly in the Democratic Republic of the Congo in November–December of 2002 an influenza H3N2 outbreak was associated with a 47% attack rate with ~1.5% mortality which was also greatest in those <5 years of age. In a recently published surveillance study conducted in Bangladesh, 28% of influenza virus culture-positive children developed pneumonia.[7]

Previous pandemics have been characterized by major changes in the genetic makeup of the virus and large portions of the population do not have pre-existing immunity to the virus. This absence of immunity is particularly common in children and young adults, while older adults may have partial immunity due to exposure to a related virus in a previous pandemic. This increased immune protection in older people that can occur to a pandemic strain of influenza virus can result in a shift in the mortality curve to a younger age during a pandemic when compared to seasonal influenza. For example, exposure to influenza A/H1 subtypes that circulated prior to 1873 appeared to have offered some protection against disease in middle-aged and older adults during the 1918 pandemic where the highest mortality rate occurred in young adults.[8]

The combination of a large number of susceptible people and a virus that is easily transmitted between people are classic features of all pandemics. The transmissibility of the virus is measured by the average number of individuals infected by an individual who already contracted the virus. Typically in seasonal influenza the reproduction number "R" is <2 which means that on average one infected person infects <2 additional people. In a pandemic, the R value is often, but not always, >2 and has been estimated to range from 1.5–5.5 in previous pandemics.[9–15] The attack rate of the virus is determined by the percentage of the population that becomes infected with the virus and is always higher for pandemic than seasonal influenza. Typically the attack rate for seasonal influenza is 5–15%, while for pandemics the attack rate is 20–50%. Once a pandemic virus enters a community via one or more infected people, the virus will spread throughout the community over a 4–8 week period. The spread of the virus occurs at different times around the world often over several years (Fig. 4). These pandemic waves can start at any time of the year, but typically are most intense during the fall and winter seasons in temperate climates and episodic but year-round in tropical climates. Usually the first wave is less intense than the second wave (most pandemics have at least two waves and some have as many as four). Seasonal viruses can circulate simultaneously with the pandemic virus adding to the burden of disease. The impact of pandemics is believed to be greater in developing countries than in developed countries, but documentation of this is lacking.[16]

During the past three centuries there have been at least 10 pandemics. A distinctive feature of pandemics is the rapid spread of disease

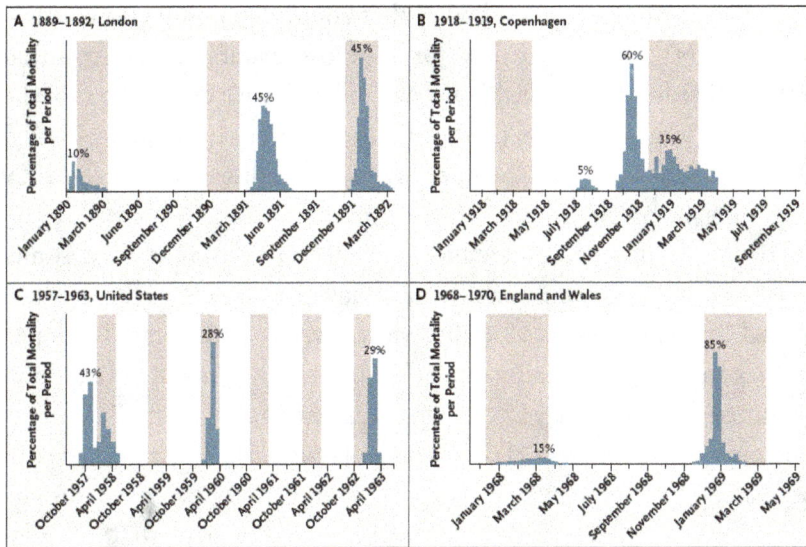

Fig. 4. The mortality distributions and periodic waves of illness noted in various cities/countries during the last four influenza pandemics occurring prior to the 2009 pandemic. The proportion of the total influenza-associated mortality burden in each wave for each of these pandemics is shown by the blue bars and each distinct blue bar indicates a separate wave and the time of year that the wave occurred. The percentage of the total mortality that occurred in each wave is also noted. The pink shaded columns show the time of year when seasonal patterns of influenza would normally occur. The pandemic of 1889–1892 (Panel A) had a relatively mild first wave that started in the winter of 1889 followed by a more intense second wave in the spring and summer of 1891 and third wave in the winter of 1891–1892. The pandemic of 1918–1919 (Panel B) had a mild first wave during the summer of 1918 followed by a severe second wave the following winter. The pandemic of 1957–1963 (Panel C) had three moderate intensity winter waves during a five-year period. The pandemic of 1968–1970 (Panel D) had a mild first wave in the winter of 1968 followed by a more intense second wave the following winter.[8]

worldwide with the first wave typically taking 6 to 9 months. Three influenza pandemics occurred in the 20th century, each resulting in illness in approximately 20–40% of the global population. The most severe previous pandemic began in 1918 and was due to a swine H1N1 influenza virus that is different from the 2009 H1N1 virus causing the current pandemic. The 1918 virus continued to evolve genetically as it continued to circulate from 1918 into the 1950s. Approximately 30% of those >60 years of age have cross-reacting antibodies that afford them protection against the 2009 H1N1 virus. The reason for this cross-reacting immunity is that people >60 years of age have likely been infected with descendents of the 1918 H1N1 virus, that didn't circulate after 1957 (see Chapters 4 and 5 for further discussion about the lower incidence of disease due to the 2009 H1N1 virus in this age group).[17,18]

The 1918 influenza pandemic is estimated to have caused somewhere between 50–100 million deaths worldwide and most of these deaths occurred in young adults. Mortality varied widely with some developed countries reporting a mortality rate below 0.5%, while in some of the poorest countries mortality may have been as high as 8%.[19] The 1957 influenza pandemic was caused by an H2N2 virus and resulted in 1–2 million deaths worldwide. The 1968 pandemic was due to an H3N2 influenza virus and caused 700,000–1,000,000 deaths worldwide. Subsequent to 1968, new viruses containing other HA and NA types have caused disease in a limited number of humans (Fig. 5), but until the occurrence of the 2009 H1N1 strain these viruses have not been able to easily spread between people.

The 2009 pandemic was first recognized in Mexico when widespread disease due to the 2009 H1N1 virus was detected. Subsequently, the virus

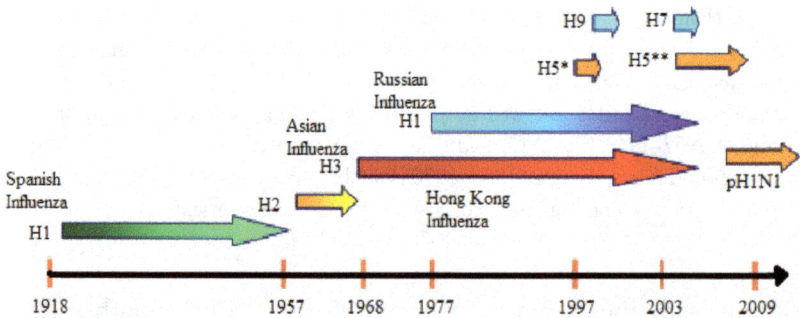

Fig. 5. Timeline of emergence of influenza A viruses in humans from early in the 20th century to the present time. This figure has been modified from a version that was on the CDC pandemic influenza website (www.pandemicflu.gov). Influenza viruses containing the H5, H7 and H9 proteins have, to date, not demonstrated the capacity to cause widespread disease in humans.

*From 1997 to 2002 the avian H5N1 virus caused disease only in animals.

**The first reported cases of avian H5N1 virus causing disease in humans occurred in 2003.

spread further into the Northern Hemisphere and then into the Southern Hemisphere. Further details of the epidemiology and demographics of the 2009 pandemic are described in Chapters 3–5.

1.1.3 *Clinical Manifestations in Epidemics and Pandemics*

> A KEY POINT: Contrary to popular belief, influenza is not just another cold. High fevers, gastrointestinal symptoms, as well as intense muscle pain can accompany the respiratory symptoms and complications are relatively common. Years ago this point was emphatically made to me when one of my professors asked me on rounds how to diagnose "the flu". I gave him a medical answer that he promptly dismissed. He then informed me that you asked the patient if they want to die, and if they said no then they do not have influenza.

Influenza is caused by a highly contagious viral infection of the respiratory tract and sometimes the gastrointestinal tract. Symptoms such as fever, cough, sore throat, body aches and marked fatigue are common and often intense. Some patients can present with diarrhea and vomiting as additional or their only symptoms. The incubation period prior to the development of symptoms is typically 1–4 days after exposure to the virus. Most people recover 3–5 days after onset of the illness. Those who are infected can shed virus for a day before symptoms appear. They usually stop being infectious within a day of resolution of their fever, but in some instances they can be infectious for 10 or more days. This prolonged infectious period is most often found in young children who often have high quantities of the virus in their nose and those with severely impaired immune systems may remain infectious for weeks or even months.

Globally, many millions of people are hospitalized and 250,000–500,000 people die from influenza each year. The most common serious complication is pneumonia. Influenza virus can invade the lung, causing pneumonia, but in most years this is not the most frequent complication.

13

More commonly lung infections are due to secondary bacterial pneumonias most often caused by *Streptococcus pneumoniae* or *Staphylococcus aureus*. Bacterial pneumonia usually occurs as the patient recovers from the initial influenza symptoms and the fever has abated. When the secondary bacterial lung infection develops, the patient's fever returns and breathing problems occur, including an increased respiratory rate and worsening cough. During the past decade, secondary infections due to community-acquired methicillin-resistant *S. aureus* (MRSA) have become more frequent and are now a major cause of hospitalization and death.

High levels of interferon are induced in those infected with influenza virus and this often results in symptoms of malaise, body and muscle aches. In some patients the myositis (muscle inflammation) is pronounced and causes the onset of moderate to severe muscle pain and tenderness, most often in the calves of both legs, and can result in the patient refusing to walk. Severe myositis is mainly associated with infection due to influenza B, but also occurs with influenza A.

Influenza virus or the associated secondary bacterial infections can also cause complications that affect the central nervous system, including viral or bacterial meningitis, viral encephalitis, encephalopathy (alterations in mental status without proof that it is caused by a microbe that has infected the brain) and Reye syndrome (a disease of unknown etiology occurring in children that is characterized by abnormalities of the liver and brain swelling and is associated with the use of aspirin). This last complication has largely disappeared after educational efforts were successful in getting the public to stop using aspirin for the treatment of fever.

Influenza frequently causes ear infections that are due to the virus or a subsequent secondary bacterial infection. Secondary bacterial infections can also occur in the blood, but are less common than those that occur in the lung. Other complications from influenza virus involving the heart (myocarditis), kidneys (renal insufficiency) and bone marrow (hemophagocytic syndrome) occur on rare occasion.

The 2009 pandemic was associated with many of the common clinical findings noted above. Most of those who became ill had fever, sore throat and/or cough. The incidence of gastrointestinal symptoms, including vomiting and diarrhea, varied in different populations (5–40%), but overall was more common than in most epidemic and pandemic years. Leukopenia (low white blood cell count), anemia and/or thrombocytopenia (low platelet count) were prominent features in some patients.[20]

1.1.4 *Laboratory Testing to Detect the Virus*

> A KEY POINT: During the past decade the laboratory capabilities for influenza testing have substantially advanced. Within days after the 2009 H1N1 virus was first grown in culture the genetic composition of the virus was determined and a reverse transcription-polymerase chain reaction test specific to this virus was developed that had very good sensitivity and specificity.

A number of different tests are available to diagnose influenza virus infections. Viral cultures using respiratory secretions have been available for many years, but it usually takes 3–7 days for the virus to grow in cell culture. Serologic testing has also been available for decades. While serologic testing is useful for population-based studies, it is not helpful for diagnosing individual cases of influenza since the need for acute and convalescent serum does not allow for a diagnosis to be made in a time frame that can be used to help make clinical decisions. For over a decade, rapid influenza tests done using nasopharyngeal swabs have been commercially available and can be done in a physician's office with results available within 30 minutes. These rapid tests are more sensitive in children than adults because children have higher amounts of the influenza virus in their nose. More recently, reverse transcription-polymerase chain reaction (RT-PCR) testing for influenza virus on respiratory specimens has become available in some laboratories. Depending on specimen transport and other logistical issues, results can be known within 1–2 days. The RT-PCR test can distinguish between influenza A (H1N1), A (H3N2) and B strains as well as within a particular strain type (e.g., between a seasonal H1N1 virus and the 2009 H1N1 virus) and is more sensitive than the rapid tests.

1.1.5 *Prevention and Treatment of Influenza Disease*

> A KEY POINT: A number of vaccines and drugs are available to prevent or treat influenza. However, several major issues could impact the ability to use these interventions during a pandemic including the possible development of viral resistance to all available antiviral agents and the high likelihood that demand for the vaccine initially outpaces the supply.

1.1.5.1 *Vaccines*

While a number of drugs have proven reasonably effective for treating influenza and decreasing the duration of viral shedding if given within 48 hours of onset of the illness, preventing influenza is clearly preferable to treating the disease. Methods of prevention include avoiding exposure to the virus, good hygiene and vaccination. While avoiding exposure to someone who is ill with any infectious disease is a great idea in theory, from a practical standpoint avoiding those who are ill is often difficult to achieve. This problem is particularly true for children who have a central role in the spread of influenza virus in a community because the rate of infection is particularly high in day care and school settings.

The annual use of influenza vaccine is the most effective means available to prevent influenza. Due to antigenic changes that occur in the virus HA and NA proteins, individuals remain susceptible to disease even if in previous years they had influenza or had been given the vaccine. The effectiveness of the vaccine is highest in years where the strain(s) of the virus circulating in the community are well matched to those contained in the vaccine being used in that particular year. Three different types of influenza viruses (A/H1N1, A/H3N2 and B) currently cause disease worldwide. Around February of each year, the WHO in consultation with various regulatory agencies determine the specific H1N1, H3N2 and B strains of influenza virus that will be used to make the trivalent vaccine for the next fall/winter season in the Northern Hemisphere. The decision is based on large part on the strains of influenza virus that are circulating in Asia at that time. Around September of each year, the WHO undergoes a similar process to determine which strains will be included in the vaccine to be used in the Southern Hemisphere. During the 2008–2009 influenza season, a seasonal H1N1 and a B strain caused the majority of disease in the USA (prior to the onset of the 2009 H1N1 virus outbreak in March 2009). The seasonal H1N1 strain circulating in the USA was a good match with the one in the vaccine, but the B strain was not as well matched. This mismatch resulted in the vaccine being more effective against the seasonal H1N1 strain than the B strain during the 2008–2009 influenza season. The seasonal H1N1 vaccine strain, that was part of the trivalent vaccine manufactured for the 2009–2010 season, was very different from the 2009 H1N1 virus and therefore the 2009–2010 seasonal vaccine did not provide protection against the pandemic virus. The lack of protection by the seasonal vaccine resulted in the need to produce an additional monovalent vaccine against the 2009 H1N1 virus.

Prior to 2010, annual immunization with influenza vaccine was routinely recommended by the CDC for all those 6 months to 18 years of age and those ≥ 50 years of age. The vaccine was also recommended for people 19–49 years of age with underlying conditions that increase their risk of serious complications and death due to influenza or who live in households with someone with these underlying conditions. These recommendations, if followed by everyone, meant that 85% of the US population would be vaccinated.

Although the number of people getting the vaccine has increased in recent years, a much greater percentage of the population needs to be vaccinated before influenza will stop being the leading cause of vaccine-preventable hospitalizations and deaths in developed countries. Table 3 shows the number of people recommended to receive the influenza vaccine who actually received the influenza vaccine during the 2008–2009 influenza season. Overall only about one-third of those recommended to receive the vaccine did so and vaccine coverage in minority populations was even lower. In an attempt to increase the vaccination rate in the USA, the ACIP at the February 2010 meeting expanded the seasonal influenza

Table 3. Estimated Seasonal Influenza Vaccination Coverage in the USA, by Age and Race/Ethnicity — Behavioral Risk Factor Surveillance System (BRFSS) in Selected States During the 2008-09 Season*†

Age group	Total§			White, non-Hispanic			Black, non-Hispanic			Hispanic		
	No.	%	(CI¶)	No.	%	(CI)	No.	%	(CI)	No.	%	(CI)
All age groups (≥6 mos)	31,130	32.6	(31.6–33.7)	24,865	36.7	(35.4–37.9)	1,173	24.9	(20.9–29.0)	2,536	22.0	(19.1–24.8)
6 mos–17 yrs	5,543	24.0	(21.8–26.4)	4,042	24.9	(22.5–27.5)	220	20.0	(13.0–29.4)	689	18.4	(13.5–24.5)
6–23 mos	416	40.9	(31.1–51.6)	306	37.2	(28.2–47.3)	—	—	—	—	—	—
2–4 yrs	788	32.0	(26.0–38.7)	529	39.6	(32.3–47.4)	—	—	—	118	16.1	(8.8–27.7)
5–17 yrs	4,339	20.8	(18.4–23.4)	3,207	21.0	(18.4–23.8)	175	20.5	(12.6–31.6)	521	16.8	(11.5–23.9)
18–49 yrs	9,493	22.2	(20.6–23.9)	7,052	25.3	(22.5–27.3)	414	16.8	(11.9–23.1)	1,115	14.8	(11.7–18.6)
18–49 yrs at high risk††	1,333	32.1	(27.5–37.1)	943	33.5	(28.4–39.2)	74	41.6	(26.1–58.9)	162	27.2	(17.1–40.5)
50–64 yrs	8,422	42.3	(40.1–44.5)	7,071	43.7	(41.6–45.7)	306	29.8	(22.0–38.9)	437	40.6	(31.7–50.1)
≥ 65 yrs	7,672	67.2	(65.0–69.4)	6,700	69.0	(67.1–70.9)	233	56.3	(45.0–66.9)	295	65.8	(53.1–76.6)

*Table 3 is an edited version of the table published in the CDC, "Prevention and Control of Influenza: Recommendations of the Advisory Committee on Immunization Practices (ACIP)", MMWR (2009) **58**(39): 1091–1095. The estimate given in the "all age groups" row is for the entire population, not just those for whom vaccination is recommended.

†Interviews were conducted primarily in January and February of 2009. Vaccination coverage estimates are based on vaccinations given during August–December, representing approximately 92% of all vaccinations administered during the entire season (August–March), based on the 2008 National Health Interview Survey.

¶95% confidence interval.

— Estimate unreliable due to small sample size.

††Respondents who have diabetes, heart disease or asthma.

recommendation to include everyone >6 months of age, unless there was a medical contraindication such as an allergy to eggs. The decision to expand the recommendation was based on the large percentage of the population already recommended to get the vaccine, the simplicity of an age-based recommendation and the experiences in Ontario, Canada, where a universal influenza vaccination has been shown to increase the vaccination rate and be cost-effective.[21]

During most epidemic years, disease due to influenza virus usually peaks sometime between January and March in the Northern Hemisphere. However, in some years, the peak occurs as early as November or as late as April. While it is optimal to get the vaccine early in the fall, vaccination as late as March can be protective. During the past decade seasonal influenza vaccine use has increased around the globe with >70 countries recommending that the vaccine be used in healthcare workers (HCWs) and/or various high-risk populations (Table 4).

Table 4. The Use of Seasonal Influenza Vaccine in Various WHO Regions, 2008*

WHO region	Number (%) of Countries in the Region Providing Seasonal Influenza Vaccine	Children Included in the Seasonal Influenza Program	Older Adults Included in the Seasonal Influenza Program	High-Risk Groups Included in the Seasonal Influenza Program
Africa	2 (4%)		1	
Americas	35 (97%)	29	35	31
Eastern Mediterranean	7 (33%)			5
Europe	26 (49%)	6	13	20
South-East Asia	2 (18%)		1	2
Western Pacific	7 (26%)	1	4	4
Total	71 (37%)	20	37	50

*Adapted from a slide presentation, "Seasonal Influenza Vaccination: Plan to Update the WHO Position Paper", by Dr. Philippe Duclos at the SAGE April 14, 2010 meeting (http://www.who.int/immunization/sage/previous_october2009/en/index1.html).

There are currently two kinds of influenza vaccine available — a trivalent inactivated (killed) influenza virus vaccine (TIV) that contains H1N1, H3N2 and B virus strains, and a live-attenuated virus vaccine (LAIV) containing the same three virus strains. While TIV contains inactivated dead virus, LAIV has been genetically altered so that the live virus can grow at temperatures found in human nasal cavities (32–33°C), but not at temperatures found in internal organs such as the lung (>37°C). TIV is given as an intramuscular injection, while LAIV is administered by spraying the vaccine into the nose. TIV is Food and Drug Administration (FDA) approved for those 6 months and older and LAIV is approved for those 2–49 years of age. TIV is approved for use in healthy people and those with chronic illnesses. LAIV is currently FDA-licensed only for healthy people.

A large number of studies involving many thousands of children and adults indicate that these influenza vaccines are effective in preventing illness. Studies suggest that LAIV is more effective than TIV in children ≤5 years of age.[22] In adults who have been previously vaccinated, TIV appears to be more effective.[23] The effectiveness of the vaccine varies year to year, but overall averages 75%. The effectiveness of the vaccine in a given year is dependent on how well matched the vaccine strains are to the viruses circulating in the area and also on the age of those being vaccinated.[24] Vaccine effectiveness is 70–90% in healthy people <65 years of age, but only 30–40% in the frail elderly. Overall, the vaccine is 50–60% effective in preventing hospitalization and ~80% effective in preventing death (presentation by Dr. John Andrus, Pan American Health Organization (PAHO) Immunization Meeting, Costa Rica, August 24–26, 2009).

Influenza vaccines are associated with relatively few adverse effects. For TIV, low grade fever is most common in those less than two years (10–35% of recipients), and occurs primarily 6 to 24 hours after vaccination. Local reactions are infrequent in children <13 years, while they occur in ~10% of adolescents and adults. Worldwide, most formulations of TIV still contain egg protein (recently in the USA and a few other countries most of the production of influenza vaccine has been changing to cell culture rather than eggs) and gelatin and should generally not be used in those who are allergic to these proteins. People with a history of Guillain–Barré syndrome (GBS), a disease that results in weakness of muscles that usually begins in the lower extremities and ascends upwards, are not recommended to receive influenza vaccine. The most common side effect of LAIV is nasal congestion. Many people mistakenly believe that LAIV can cause influenza, but the LAIV virus is genetically engineered so that it cannot do this. Furthermore, studies show that flu-like symptoms are no more common in those who received LAIV than those who did not.

1.1.5.2 *Antivirals*

Two classes of influenza antiviral drugs are currently licensed in most countries: adamantanes (amantadine [Symmetrel^R] and rimantadine [Flumadine^R]) and neuraminidase inhibitors (oseltamivir [Tamiflu^R] and zanamivir [Relenza^R]). These drugs have been shown to reduce the severity and shorten the duration of influenza illness by one to two days if treatment is started within 48 hours of onset of symptoms. These drugs also decrease the amount of influenza virus in the nose, thereby reducing the chance that an infected person will pass the virus to others. For seasonal influenza, treatment with antiviral therapy is recommended for any child or adult at high risk for complications from influenza or for anyone with influenza in whom it may be useful to reduce the duration of symptoms. While the use of influenza vaccine is clearly the preferred method for preventing influenza, these drugs can also be used to prevent illness in an unvaccinated person who is exposed to someone with influenza (Table 5).

Amantadine and rimantadine are given orally and work by blocking viral replication of some strains of influenza type A. Disadvantages of amantadine and rimantadine include: (1) emergence of resistance in most circulating strains of influenza A/H3N2, (2) lack of activity against influenza type B, and (3) the occurrence of reversible central nervous system (CNS) side effects including nervousness, lightheadedness, difficulty with concentration and, rarely, tremors or seizures.

The neuraminidase inhibitors oseltamivir and zanamivir work by interfering with the release of viral particles from the surface of infected

Table 5. Persons for Whom Antiviral Treatment and Prophylaxis Should be Considered During Periods When Seasonal Influenza is in the Community

Treatment*

Persons for whom antiviral treatment should be considered include those:

- hospitalized with laboratory-confirmed influenza (limited data suggests benefit even for persons whose antiviral treatment is initiated >48 hours after illness onset);
- with laboratory-confirmed influenza pneumonia;
- with laboratory-confirmed influenza and bacterial co-infection;
- with laboratory-confirmed influenza infection who are at higher risk for influenza complications; and
- presenting for medical care with laboratory-confirmed influenza within 48 hours of influenza illness onset and who want to decrease the duration or severity of their symptoms and transmission of influenza to others at higher risk for complications.

Chemoprophylaxis[†]

Persons for whom antiviral chemoprophylaxis should be considered include those:

- persons at high risk for severe disease due to influenza during the 2 weeks after influenza vaccination (after the second dose for children aged <9 years who have not previously been vaccinated);*
- persons at high risk for whom influenza vaccine is contraindicated;
- family members or healthcare providers who are unvaccinated and are likely to have ongoing, close exposure to persons at high risk or to unvaccinated persons or infants aged <6 months;
- persons at high risk, their family members and close contacts, and healthcare workers, when circulating strains of influenza virus in the community are not well matched with vaccine strains;
- persons with immune deficiencies or those who might not respond to vaccination (e.g., persons infected with human immunodeficiency virus or with other immunosuppressed conditions, or who are receiving immunosuppressive medications); and
- unvaccinated staff and persons during response to an outbreak in a closed institutional setting with residents at high risk (e.g., extended-care facilities).

Adapted from the CDC publication, "Prevention and Control of Influenza: Recommendations of the Advisory Committee on Immunization Practices (ACIP)", *MMWR* (2008) **57**(RR-7): 38.

*If possible, antiviral treatment should be started within 48 hours of influenza illness onset. The effectiveness of initiating antiviral treatment >48 hours after the onset of illness has not been established in most circumstances.

[†]Influenza vaccination induces a protective immune response by two weeks after immunization and this often allows the discontinuance of chemoprophylaxis after that point.

respiratory tract cells. Oseltamivir is taken orally and until recently was approved for use only in those who are ≥ 2 years of age. In response to the 2009 pandemic, the Food and Drug Administration issued an Emergency Use Authorization for use of this drug for all ages. Oseltamivir is associated with nausea and vomiting in approximately 10% of recipients. Oseltamivir has also been shown to reduce the incidence of serious complications such as bacterial pneumonia. Zanamivir is a powder taken by inhalation through a breath-activated device and is approved for use only in those who are ≥ 7 years of age. The safety and efficacy of zanamivir in patients with chronic lung disease has not been established. Some patients with a history of asthma have experienced wheezing when given the drug, and zanamivir is generally not recommended for patients with underlying airway disease. Until recently, both neuraminidase inhibitors were effective for the treatment of influenza type A or type B if given within 48 hours of the onset of symptoms. However, during the last few years, the influenza A H1N1 strains causing non-pandemic seasonal disease have become resistant to oseltamivir, but remain susceptible to zanamivir.

When determining the timing and duration for administering influenza antiviral medications for prevention of influenza, factors related to cost, compliance and potential adverse events need to be considered. To be maximally effective as prophylaxis agents, the drugs must be taken each day for the duration of influenza activity in the community or until the person has been vaccinated and had enough time to develop immunity. Prophylactic use of these drugs should not be considered a substitute for vaccination.

The recent occurrence of oseltamivir resistance among influenza A H1N1 virus strains presents challenges for the selection of antiviral medications for treatment and chemoprophylaxis of influenza. The development of resistance provides additional reasons for clinicians to consult surveillance data to determine whether someone with acute respiratory illness is likely to have influenza and if so which strains are circulating in their community. If available, confirmatory testing with rapid diagnostic tests capable of distinguishing influenza disease caused by influenza H1N1 from H3N2 or influenza B virus can be used to guide treatment. When the specific strain of influenza virus causing disease in a patient cannot be determined, treatment with both a neuraminidase inhibitor and an adamantane should be considered unless the specific strain(s) circulating in the community are known to be sensitive to one of these drugs. Updated guidelines have been provided by the CDC about the use of antivirals for the treatment and chemoprophylaxis of influenza that take into account the problems with resistant strains.[25]

References

1. Hunt M. (2010) Influenza virus (orthmyxovirus). In: Hunt RC (ed), *Microbiology and Immunology On-line*, Chapter 13 [http://pathmicro.med.sc.edu/mhunt/flu.htm]. University of South Carolina School of Medicine, Columbia, SC.

2. Shinde V, Bridges CB, Uyeki TM *et al.* (2009) Triple-reassortant swine influenza A (H1) in humans in the United States, 2005–2009. *N Engl J Med* **360**: 2616–2625. Erratum in: *N Engl J Med* **361**: 102.

3. Belshe RB. (2009) Implications of the emergence of a novel H1 influenza virus. *N Engl J Med* **360**: 2667–2668.

4. Trifonov V, Khiabanian H, Rabadan R. (2009) Geographic dependence, surveillance, and origins of the 2009 influenza A (H1N1) virus. *N Engl J Med* **361**: 115–119.

5. Santibañez S, Fiore AE, Merlin TL, Redd S. (2009) A primer on strategies for prevention and control of seasonal and pandemic influenza. *Am J Public Health* **99**(Suppl 2): S216–224.

6. Viboud C, Alonso WJ, Simonsen L. (2006) Influenza in tropical regions. *PLoS Med* **3**: e89.

7. Brooks WA, Goswami D, Rahman M *et al.* (2010) Influenza is a major contributor to childhood pneumonia in a tropical developing country. *Pediatr Infect Dis J* **29**: 216–221.

8. Miller MA, Viboud C, Balinska M, Simonsen L. (2009) The signature features of influenza pandemics – Implications for policy. *N Engl J Med* **360**: 2595–2598.

9. Fraser C, Donnelly CA, Cauchemez S *et al.*; WHO Rapid Pandemic Assessment Collaboration. (2009) Pandemic potential of a strain of influenza A (H1N1): Early findings. *Science* **324**: 1557–1561 [Epub May 11, 2009. PubMed PMID: 19433588].

10. Longini IM Jr, Nizam A, Xu S *et al.* (2005) Containing pandemic influenza at the source. *Science* **309**: 1083–1087 [Epub 2005. PubMed PMID: 16079251].

11. Chowell G, Bettencourt LM, Johnson N *et al.* (2008) The 1918–1919 influenza pandemic in England and Wales: Spatial patterns in transmissibility and mortality impact. *Proc Biol Sci* **275**: 501–509 [PubMed PMID: 18156123; PubMed Central PMCID: PMC2596813].

12. Chowell G, Nishiura H, Bettencourt LM. (2007) Comparative estimation of the reproduction number for pandemic influenza from daily case notification data. *J R Soc Interface* **4**: 155–166 [PubMed PMID: 17254982; PubMed Central PMCID: PMC2358966].

13. Chowell G, Ammon CE, Hengartner NW, Hyman JM. (2006) Estimation of the reproductive number of the Spanish flu epidemic in Geneva, Switzerland. *Vaccine* **24**: 6747–6750 [Epub Jun 5, 2006. PubMed PMID: 16782243].

14. Andreasen V, Viboud C, Simonsen L. (2008) Epidemiologic characterization of the 1918 influenza pandemic summer wave in Copenhagen: Implications for pandemic control strategies. *J Infect Dis* **197**: 270–278 [PubMed PMID: 18194088; PubMed Central PMCID: PMC2674012].

15. Mills CE, Robins JM, Lipsitch M. (2004) Transmissibility of 1918 pandemic influenza. *Nature* **432**: 904–906 [PubMed PMID: 15602562].

16. Considerations for assessing the severity of an influenza pandemic. (2009) *Wkly Epidemiol Rec* **84**: 197–202.

17. Krause JC, Tumpey MT, Huffman CJ *et al.* (2010) Naturally occurring human monoclonal antibodies neutralize both 1918 and 2009 pandemic influenza A (H1N1) viruses. *J Virol* **84**: 3127.

18. Xu R, Ekiert DC, Krause JC *et al.* (2010) Structural basis of preexisting immunity to the 2009 H1N1 pandemic influenza virus. *Science* **328**: 357–360.

19. Murray CJ, Lopez AD, Chin B *et al.* (2006) Estimation of potential global pandemic influenza mortality on the basis of vital registry data from the 1918–20 pandemic: A quantitative analysis. *Lancet* **368**: 2211–2218.

20. Peiris JS, Poon LL, Guan Y. (2009) Emergence of a novel swine-origin influenza A virus (S-OIV) H1N1 virus in humans. *J Clin Virol* **45**: 169–173.

21. Sander B, Kwong JC, Bauch CT *et al.* (2010) Economic appraisal of Ontario's Universal Influenza Immunization Program: A cost-utility analysis. *PLoS Med* **7**: e1000256.

22. Belshe RB, Edwards KM, Vesikari T *et al.*; CAIV-T Comparative Efficacy Study Group. (2007) Live attenuated versus inactivated influenza vaccine in infants and young children. *N Engl J Med* **356**: 685–696.

23. Wang Z, Tobler S, Roayaei J, Eick A. (2009) Live attenuated or inactivated influenza vaccines and medical encounters for respiratory illnesses among US military personnel. *JAMA* **301**: 945–953.

24. Glezen WP. (2008) Clinical practice: Prevention and treatment of seasonal influenza. *N Engl J Med* **359**: 2579–2585.

25. CDC Health Advisory. (2008) CDC issues interim recommendations for the use of influenza antiviral medications in the setting of oseltamivir resistance among circulating influenza A (H1N1) viruses, 2008–09 Influenza Season [http://www2a.cdc.gov/HAN/Archivesys/ViewMsgV.asp?alertnum=00279, updated December 19].

Chapter 2

Planning for a Pandemic

"Avian influenza is not a challenge. It is a predicament of extraordinary proportions. Doctors must say this loudly and repeatedly. Presently, we are largely silent. As the *Lancet* wrote after the 1918 influenza pandemic, if only we had acted earlier with a 'collective health conscience', many millions of lives could have been saved. Today, we are repeating the same mistakes of a century ago."

The Lancet (2006) **367**: 1550

2.1 Pandemic Planning

> A KEY POINT: During the 2009 pandemic, many lives were saved because we planned well. Other lives were lost because we did not plan well enough.

2.1.1 *Development of a Pandemic Plan*

The periodic nature of previous pandemics left little doubt amongst scientists and public health officials that another pandemic would occur in the future and this prediction led many countries to develop contingency plans to deal with the next pandemic. In large part, these plans were country-specific, but there were various coordinating efforts that occurred between countries.

2.1.2 *Worldwide*

The degree of pandemic planning across the globe varied substantially in different countries. In general, developing countries had done far less planning than developed countries. One of the mechanisms that was available to help deal with this problem was the Global Health Security Initiative which is an informal, international partnership created in 2001 by Canada, the European Union, France, Germany, Italy, Japan, Mexico, the United Kingdom and the USA to strengthen global health preparedness and responsiveness to threats of biological, chemical and nuclear terrorism as well as pandemic influenza (http://www.ghsi.ca/english/index.asp). The Global Health Security Initiative was created to address current health issues including global health security, and was not intended to replace, overlap or duplicate existing networks. The WHO serves as an expert advisor to the Global Health Security Initiative and a great deal of this group's activity during the past three years had focused on pandemic flu preparedness, including:

- Joint cooperation in procuring vaccines and antibiotics.
- Rapid testing, research in variations of vaccines, and coordinating respective regulatory frameworks for the development of vaccines.
- Further supporting the WHO's disease surveillance network and efforts to develop a coordinated strategy for disease outbreak containment.
- Sharing emergency preparedness and response plans, including contact lists, and considering joint training and planning.
- Developing a process for international collaboration on risk assessment and management and a common language for risk communication.
- Improving linkages among laboratories, including level four laboratories, in those countries which have them.

Once the 2009 pandemic was declared, two Global Health Security Initiative Special Ministerial Meetings were held in September and December 2009. These meetings helped the Global Health Security Initiative work in collaboration with the WHO to improve the access of developing and developed countries to H1N1 vaccines, antiviral drugs

and other medical supplies, monitor vaccine safety, and coordinate effective public health and healthcare measures to mitigate the impact of the
pandemic.

2.1.3 *United States of America*

In the USA, pandemic planning efforts first started in 1978 and greatly
intensified during the past decade. These plans were designed to provide guidance to help mitigate the impact of the next pandemic and
identify issues that needed to be addressed at federal, state and local
levels — in both the public and private sectors. The potential impact
of the next influenza pandemic in the USA was modeled in 1999 by the
CDC (Table 6).[26] Based on previous pandemics, hospitalization and mortality rates were estimated to increase 2–6-fold compared to that seen
in epidemic years. The results of this modeling were sensitive to both
the attack rate and virulence of the virus. Further modeling was done
in 2005 to estimate the impact of a moderate versus severe pandemic
on various parameters including the number of people who would seek
medical care, be hospitalized and die (Table 7). Additionally, clear definitions for the staging of a possible pandemic (Fig. 6), the criteria used to
define the severity of a pandemic (Fig. 7) and interventions that should

Table 6. The Impact of a Typical Epidemic Influenza Season Compared to a
Pandemic Influenza Season

Annual Epidemic	Pandemic
~36,000 deaths in the USA	89,000 to 207,000 USA deaths
~90% in the elderly	younger ages hit harder
~114,000 hospitalizations	~314,000 to 734,000 hospitalizations
highest rate in those <24 mth of age	highest rate can be in any age group
Infection in 5–15% of population	Infection in 20–50% of the population
Cost to economy ~$12 billion/yr*	Cost to economy $71 to 167 billion*

Adapted from CDC pandemic modeling done in 1999.[26]
*In 1999 dollars.

29

Table 7. The Impact of the Severity of a Pandemic on Medical Resources that will be Needed and Medical Outcomes

Characteristic	Moderate Severity Based on 1957 & 1968 Pandemics*	High Severity Based on 1918 Pandemic*
Illness	90 million (30%)	90 million (30%)
Outpatient medical care	45 million (50%)	45 million (50%)
Hospitalization	865,000	9,900,000
ICU care	128,750	1,485,000
Mechanical ventilation	64,875	742,500
Deaths	209,000	1,903,000

Adapted from a presentation at the Health and Human Services Pandemic Influenza planning meeting in October 2005.
*The 1957 and 1968 influenza pandemics were considered to be of moderate severity while the 1918 pandemic was very severe.

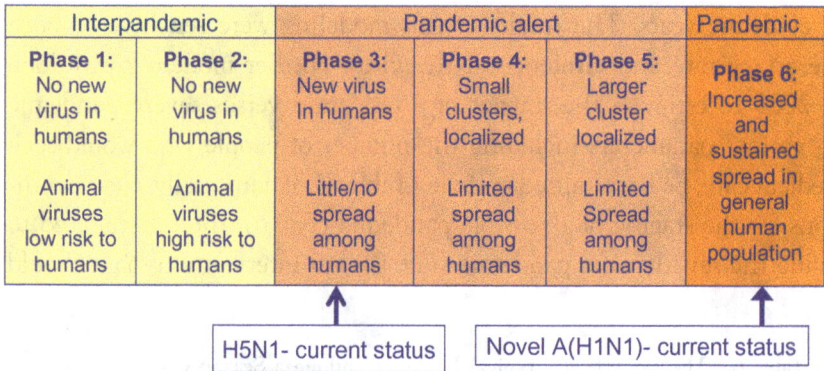

Interpandemic		Pandemic alert			Pandemic
Phase 1: No new virus in humans	**Phase 2:** No new virus in humans	**Phase 3:** New virus In humans	**Phase 4:** Small clusters, localized	**Phase 5:** Larger cluster localized	**Phase 6:** Increased and sustained spread in general human population
Animal viruses low risk to humans	Animal viruses high risk to humans	Little/no spread among humans	Limited spread among humans	Limited Spread among humans	

H5N1- current status   Novel A(H1N1)- current status

Fig. 6. The definitions used to describe the various stages that occur prior to and at the time a pandemic is underway (http://www.cdc.gov/flu/pandemic/phases.htm). The arrows note the highest pandemic phase reached by the avian H5N1 and the 2009 H1N1 influenza viruses. The avian H5N1 virus phase 3 alert was issued by the WHO in 2003, but because this virus has not acquired the ability to spread easily between humans, further progression to a higher pandemic alert level has not occurred. In contrast, the 2009 H1N1 virus phase 3, 4 and 5 alerts were issued by the WHO in April 2009 and by June 11, 2009, the WHO changed the alert level to phase 6 due to the rapid transmission of the virus around the globe.

Case Fatality Ratio		Projected Number of Deaths US Population, 2006
≥2.0%	Category 5	≥1,800,000
1.0 - <2.0%	Category 4	900,000 - <1,800,000
0.5 - <1.0%	Category 3	450,000 - <900,000
0.1 - <0.5%	Category 2	90,000 - <450,000
<0.1%	Category 1	<90,000

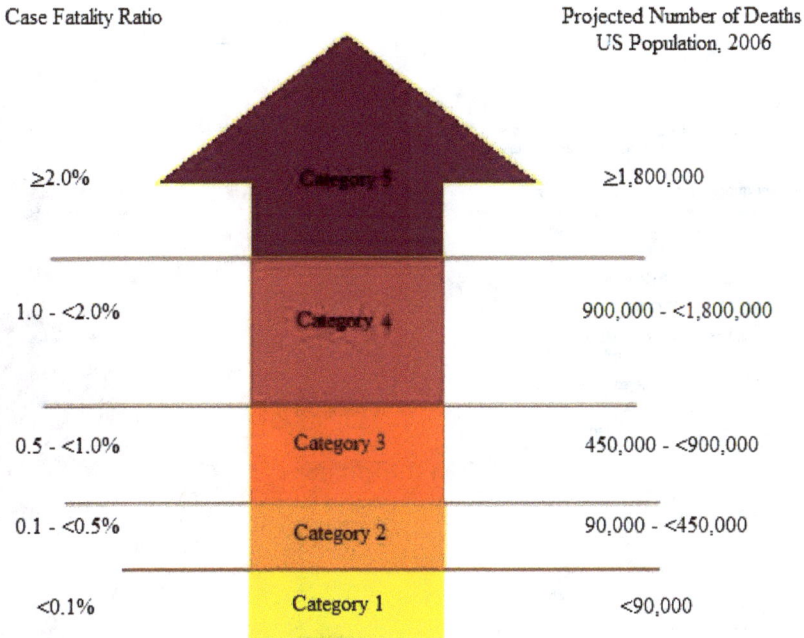

Fig. 7. The criteria used to define the severity of a pandemic (http://pandemicflu.gov/ professional/community/commitigation.html#XV, Fig. 4).

be considered once a pandemic was underway were developed by the CDC (Fig. 8).

Preparedness for a pandemic, a process that can take many years, requires the establishment of infrastructure and capacity to detect a new pandemic virus, prevent infection in as many people as possible and treat those who become ill. Based in part on the concern about whether the avian H5N1 virus would soon cause a pandemic, the USA Department of Health and Human Services made available for public comment a draft of the National Pandemic Influenza Preparedness Plan in 2004.[27] Thereafter, President George W. Bush announced the National Strategy for Pandemic Influenza (The Strategy) on November 1, 2005.[28] The Strategy noted that the federal government played a pivotal role in developing the Strategy and providing the financing to

	Pandemic Severity		
	Category 1	Category 2 & 3	Category 4&5
Home			
Voluntary isolation of ill at home (adults and children); combine with use of antiviral treatment as available and indicated	Recommend	Recommend	Recommend
Voluntary quarantine of household			
Members in homes with ill persons (adults and children); consider combining with antiviral prophylaxis if effective, feasible, and quantities sufficient.	Generally not Recommended	Consider	Recommend
Workplace/Community			
Adult social distancing			
-decrease number of social contacts (e.g., encourage teleconferences, alternative to face-to-face meetings)	Generally not recommended	Consider	Recommend
-increase distance between persons (e.g., reduce density in public transit, workplace)	Generally not recommended	Consider	Recommend
-modify, postpone, or cancel selected public gatherings to promote social distance (e.g., stadium events, theater performances)	Generally not recommended	Consider	Recommend
-modify workplace schedules and practices (e.g., telework, staggered shifts)	Generally not recommended	Consider	Recommend
School			
Child social distancing			
-dismissal of students from schools and school-based activities, and closure of child care programs	Generally not recommended	Consider: ≤ 4 weeks	Recommend: ≤ 12 weeks
-reduce out-of-school contacts and community mixing	Generally not recommended	Consider: ≤ 4 weeks	Recommend: ≤ 12 weeks

Fig. 8. Community intervention strategies that should be deployed based on the severity of a pandemic (http://pandemicflu.gov/professional/community/commitigation.html#XV, Table 2). The definitions for pandemic severity categories are noted in Fig. 7.

implement the plan, but putting the plan into practice would for the most part need to occur at the state and community level. The Strategy made clear that an effective coordinated international response was also crucial. The Strategy contains three pillars: (1) preparedness and communication; (2) surveillance and detection; and (3) response and containment.

The federal, state and local governments, healthcare providers, the private sector and private citizens all have important and interdependent roles in preparing for, responding to and recovering from a pandemic. State and local governments are primarily responsible for detecting and responding to disease outbreaks and implementing measures to minimize the consequences of an outbreak. CDC guidelines were made available to local communities to provide guidance on prevention and treatment interventions that should be used based on the severity of the pandemic (Fig. 8). The federal government's role was felt to include providing some of the response personnel and expertise, response materials, diagnostic reference services and testing support, and funding for certain response activities. It was anticipated that a severe pandemic could overwhelm state and local capabilities and that federal agencies might be called upon to provide additional support, but even those resources could be overwhelmed at the peak of a pandemic.

The private sector, including those entities involved in critical infrastructure, also has a major role in a pandemic. Unlike some catastrophic events, an influenza pandemic will not directly affect the physical infrastructure of an organization. However, a pandemic could potentially threaten critical infrastructure by impacting an organization's human resources by causing illness in essential personnel from the workplace for prolonged periods. Critical infrastructure encompasses those systems and assets that are so vital that their incapacity would have a debilitating impact on the nation's security, economy, public health or safety. Therefore, it is crucial that organizations anticipate the potential impact of a pandemic on personnel and ensure that reasonable measures are in place to help protect the health of personnel.

The success or failure of community-based infection control measures ultimately depends upon the acts of individuals, and the collective response of all Americans and others around the world. The Strategy notes that: (1) individuals will, in general, respond to a pandemic and to public health interventions in ways that they perceive to be congruent with their interests and instinct for self-preservation, (2) public health authorities should tailor their risk communication campaigns and interventions accordingly, and (3) institutions in danger of becoming overwhelmed will rely on the volunteerism and sense of civic and humanitarian duty of individuals whose talents and skills are crucial to the Nation's medical, economic and social responses to a pandemic.

2.1.3.1 *Assumptions upon which the Strategy was based*

> A KEY POINT: Given that the epidemiology of each pandemic differs in significant ways, many assumptions had to be made as the pandemic plan was devised. For the 2009 pandemic many of these assumptions were on target, but there were some major surprises.

Pandemics are unpredictable. While history offers useful benchmarks, there is no way to accurately predict the characteristics and potential impact of a particular pandemic. Nevertheless, assumptions must be made to facilitate planning efforts. The Strategy was based on the following assumptions (the italicized text discusses instances where these assumptions were substantially off target [also see Chapter 6]).

1. Susceptibility to the pandemic influenza virus would be universal. *Unlike the younger age groups, a substantial percentage of adults >60 years of age had cross-reacting antibodies to the 2009 H1N1. These cross-reacting antibodies provided this age group with significant protection against developing disease which resulted in a marked downward shift in the age of those who were hospitalized and died.*[29]
2. Efficient and sustained person-to-person transmission signals that a pandemic is imminent.
3. The clinical disease attack rate would be ~30% in the overall population during the pandemic. Illness rates would be highest among school-age children (~40%), decline with age and average ~20% in working adults during a community outbreak.
4. Some people would be infected but not develop clinically significant symptoms, but asymptomatic or minimally symptomatic individuals can transmit infection and develop immunity to subsequent infection.
5. In previous pandemics, approximately half of those who became ill sought care. With the availability of effective antiviral medications for treatment, this percentage might be higher in the next pandemic.

6. Rates of serious illness, hospitalization and death depend on the virulence of the pandemic virus and differ by a log order of magnitude between more and less severe scenarios. Risk groups for severe and fatal infection cannot be predicted with certainty but are likely to include infants, the elderly, pregnant women, and persons with chronic or immunosuppressive medical conditions. *Many elderly people had cross-reacting antibodies against this 2009 H1N1 virus and this immunity resulted in a lower attack rate in this age group. The actual number of deaths in the elderly were ~80% less than seen with seasonal influenza, but the number of deaths in children were ~500% greater than seen in seasonal influenza (statement made by Dr. Anne Schuchat, Director of the National Center for Immunization and Respiratory Diseases, at the ACIP meeting on February 24, 2010). As was predicted in the Strategy, pregnant women also had a very high rate of hospitalization and death. A planning meeting was held in 2008 to obtain input from experts regarding the clinical and public health issues that would likely arise in pregnant women during a pandemic.*[30]

7. Rates of absenteeism depend on the severity of the pandemic. In a severe pandemic, absenteeism due to illness, the need to care for sick family members and fear of infection may reach 40% during the peak weeks of a community outbreak. Certain public health measures (closing schools, quarantining household contacts of infected individuals), if utilized, would likely increase rates of absenteeism.

8. The typical incubation period between infection and onset of symptoms for influenza is approximately two days.

9. Persons who become ill can transmit infection for up to one day before the onset of illness and the risk of transmission will be greatest during the first two days of illness. Children will play a major role in transmission of infection as their illness rates are likely to be higher, they shed more virus over a longer time, and they control their secretions less well.

10. On average, infected persons will transmit infection to approximately two other people. *Between various communities the average number of people who are secondarily infected by each person (i.e., the reproductive*

[R] *value) value varied widely with some places reporting R values as high as 3.3 and other places <2. The R value appeared to be impacted by the age of the population studied and the population density.*[31–33]

11. Pandemic waves will last 6–8 weeks in affected communities.

12. Multiple waves (periods during which community outbreaks occur across the country) of illness will occur with each wave lasting 2–3 months. Historically, the largest waves have occurred in the fall and winter, but the seasonality of a pandemic cannot be predicted with certainty. *During the summer of 2009, the incidence of disease was higher than seen at the same time of year during epidemic years in the USA and other Northern Hemisphere countries. A second wave did occur in the fall and winter of 2009–2010 in these countries and this wave had the greatest health impact in most instances.*

2.1.3.2 *Implementing the pandemic plan strategy*

> A KEY POINT: Not surprisingly, the goals of the implementation plan that needed to be achieved early in the pandemic were less successful than those that occurred later on.

Beginning in 2005, the US government took a historic series of actions, domestically and internationally, to plan for the next pandemic including authorizing a $7.1 billion budget that was used over multiple years to support pandemic preparedness, establishing an International Partnership on Avian and Pandemic Influenza, and initiating the first Cabinet-level exercise to assess the federal government response to a naturally occurring threat. The goals of the federal government response to a pandemic were to:

1. Stop, slow or otherwise limit the spread of a pandemic to the USA. *This goal was not successfully met.*

2. Limit the domestic spread of a pandemic, and mitigate disease, suffering and death. *This goal was only partially achieved during the first and second*

wave. The biggest impediment was an inadequate supply of vaccine at the time the first and second pandemic wave occurred in most countries.

3. Sustain infrastructure and mitigate impact to the economy and the functioning of society. *This goal was, for the most part, successfully achieved.*

In addition to coordinating a comprehensive and timely national response, the federal government had primary responsibility for certain critical functions, including:

- The support of containment efforts overseas and limitation of the arrival of a pandemic to our shores.
- Guidance related to protective measures that should be taken.
- Modifications to the law and regulations to facilitate the national pandemic response.
- Modifications to monetary policy to mitigate the economic impact of a pandemic on communities and the nation as a whole.
- Procurement and distribution of vaccine and antiviral medications.
- The acceleration of research and development of vaccines and therapies during the outbreak.

A more detailed discussion of the reasons why some of these goals and objectives were accomplished and others were not can be found in Chapter 6 and consideration is given to what can be done to better prepare for the next pandemic in Chapter 7.

References

26. Meltzer MI, Cox NJ, Fukuda K. (1999) The economic impact of pandemic influenza in the United States: Priorities for intervention. *Emerg Infect Dis* **5**: 659–671.
27. US Department of Health & Human Services. (2004) National Pandemic Influenza Preparedness Plan [http://www.hhs.gov/pandemicflu/plan].
28. US Department of Health & Human Services. (2005) National Strategy for Pandemic Influenza [http://www.flu.gov/professional/federal/index.html#national].

29. Hancock K, Veguilla V, Lu X *et al.* (2009) Cross-reactive antibody responses to the 2009 pandemic H1N1 influenza virus. *N Engl J Med* **361**: 1945–1952.

30. Rasmussen SA, Jamieson DJ, Macfarlane K *et al.*; Pandemic Influenza and Pregnancy Working Group. (2009) Pandemic influenza and pregnant women: Summary of a meeting of experts. *Am J Public Health* **Suppl 2**: S248–S254.

31. Lessler J, Reich NG, Cummings DA; New York City Department of Health and Mental Hygiene Swine Influenza Investigation Team, Nair HP, Jordan HT, Thompson N. (2009) Outbreak of 2009 pandemic influenza A (H1N1) at a New York City school. *N Engl J Med* **361**: 2628–2636.

32. Miller E, Hoschler K, Hardelid P *et al.* (2010) Incidence of 2009 pandemic influenza A H1N1 infection in England: A cross-sectional serological study. *Lancet* **375**: 1100–1108.

33. Dietz K. (1993) The estimation of the basic reproduction number for infectious diseases. *Stat Methods Med Res* **2**: 23–41.

Chapter 3

A Pandemic is Imminent:
The First Wave Begins
(March through May 2009)

"The WHO pandemic phases are based on the geographical spread of a pandemic virus and are intended as a global call to countries to increase their alertness and readiness. However, within each phase, countries may find it useful to assess the specific severity parameters of a pandemic at the national or regional level, as such assessments can be used to efficiently target and scale the use of limited resources and interventions aimed at lowering pandemic-associated morbidity and mortality."

WHO Weekly Epidemiological Record, May 29, 2009

3.1 An Imminent Pandemic: Phases 3–5

A KEY POINT: Most experts had predicted that the next pandemic would start in Asia and the fact that the outbreak due to the 2009 H1N1 virus began in Mexico was a major surprise. The initial worldwide response to this outbreak did not result in a substantial containment of the virus, but did have a marked detrimental effect on Mexico's economy including an almost complete shutdown of its tourism industry. Furthermore, many local governments and communities throughout the world had done minimal planning until the 2009 pandemic actually occurred. In large part, this was because they already had other pressing healthcare problems and did not have the additional resources needed to deal with a problem that was not immediately impacting them.

3.1.1 *An Influenza Outbreak Begins in Mexico and Spreads to the United States and Other Countries*

An outbreak of influenza-like illness in Veracruz, Mexico, was reported to the WHO on April 12, 2009. By April 23, there were more than 854 cases of pneumonia in Mexico City with 59 deaths and the 2009 H1N1 virus was confirmed in several patients.[34] On April 24, the WHO reported that in the Federal District of Mexico, surveillance had begun to pick up cases of influenza-like illness as early as March 18, 2009, and the WHO declared a public health event of international concern. In San Luis Potosi, in central Mexico, 24 cases of influenza-like illness had been detected, with three deaths reported, and from Mexicali, near the USA border, there were four cases of influenza-like illness reported. On April 29, the WHO declared pandemic phase 4 based on the sustained community transmission in Mexico (see Chapter 2, Fig. 6). Subsequent analysis of the genetic sequence of the 2009 H1N1 virus showed that the initial transmission to humans occurred several months before the outbreak was recognized.[35]

The initial definition of a suspected case of 2009 H1N1 virus infection was any hospitalized patient with severe acute respiratory illness, but this definition was expanded on May 1 to include any person with acute respiratory illness defined as fever with either sore throat or cough. On May 11 the case definition for a suspected case was further refined to include any person with fever, cough and headache (or irritability in children <5 years of age) plus one or more of the following symptoms: rhinorrhea, nasal congestion, prostration, myalgias, arthralgias, chest pain and abdominal pain. A laboratory-confirmed case of 2009 H1N1 virus infection was defined as any person in whom a respiratory specimen tested positive using RT-PCR.

By the end of May there were 5,337 confirmed cases of the 2009 H1N1 virus in Mexico. The overall case rate in the population was 5/100,000, and 42%, 32%, 24% and 2% of the cases occurred in those <15, 15–29, 30–60 and >60 years of age, respectively. The fact that the incidence of disease was very low in those >60 years of age was surprising. Subsequent studies showed that serum cross-reacting antibodies occurred in 0% of those <19 years of age, <10% of those 19–60 years of age and 33% of those >60 years of age. From a genetic standpoint the HA of this virus was somewhat similar to the HA of the H1N1 viruses that circulated from the 1918 through the late 1940s and also provided a possible explanation for why the incidence of disease was inversely related to age.[17,18,29] The relatively large number of non-elderly people requiring hospitalization during this initial outbreak in Mexico caused substantial concern among many public health officials around the globe that this was the start of a potentially severe pandemic.

The first two cases of 2009 H1N1 virus infection in the USA were detected in Southern California between April 15–17, 2009. On April 24, the USA government reported seven confirmed human cases of the 2009 H1N1 virus (five in California and two in Texas) and nine suspected cases. All seven confirmed cases had mild influenza-like illness, with only one requiring brief hospitalization. Many additional cases were reported in California and Texas during the next couple of weeks, and on April 29 the WHO declared that the pandemic was in phase 5 since there was now sustained community transmission in two countries (Mexico and the USA). During this time five other countries also reported a small number of confirmed cases.

3.1.2 *Worldwide*

From the beginning, the WHO had clearly and consistently advised against restrictions of regular travel or closure of borders. The WHO also noted that there was no risk of contracting the quadravalent 2009 H1N1 virus from consumption of well-cooked pork or pork products. Despite this advice, early on in the pandemic many countries advised against travel to Mexico, and in Egypt over 300,000 pigs were slaughtered despite the WHO guidance. Additionally, a clear consensus on what the designated name of the virus that caused the 2009 pandemic should be was never achieved. Several names that were used at the beginning of the pandemic and some of the problems associated with these names included:

1. Swine influenza virus — This name was not specific enough since previous outbreaks and pandemics had been caused by other influenza viruses

that contained swine genetic material. Additionally, the pork industry objected to the name since they were concerned the public would incorrectly assume that people could get infected with the virus due to eating pork products.

2. Novel influenza virus — This name also was not specific enough since pandemics are caused by influenza viruses that are substantially different from previous influenza viruses and it is these novel features of the virus that result in most or all of the population having no immunity to the virus.

3. 2009 H1N1 pandemic virus — Most articles use this name or the shortened version, "2009 H1N1 virus" (the designation used in this book), since it made it easier for the public to understand that this virus caused the 2009 pandemic.

The Strategic Advisory Group of Experts on Immunization (SAGE) was established by the WHO Director-General in 1999 as the principal advisory group to the WHO on vaccines and immunization issues. SAGE is comprised of 15 members from around the world who serve in a voluntary capacity and represent a broad range of disciplines in fields that include epidemiology, public health, vaccinology, pediatrics, internal medicine, infectious diseases, immunology, drug regulation, program management, immunization delivery and healthcare administration. On April 29, 2009, the WHO formed several ad hoc committees to provide advice to the Director-General, Dr. Margaret Chan, about steps that needed to be taken to prepare for what was now believed to be an imminent pandemic. One of these groups, the Ad Hoc Policy Advisory SAGE Working Group on Influenza A (H1N1) Vaccines, consisted of two SAGE members and various other people with specific expertise related to pandemic influenza, vaccine safety, regulatory issues and other areas. The working group held a number of conference calls and provided input to SAGE on issues related to the potential use of a pandemic vaccine. This was done in preparation for a meeting in Geneva on July 7, 2009, when SAGE would meet to advise the WHO Director-General on how a pandemic vaccine could most effectively be used (see Chapter 4 for the deliberations that occurred at that meeting).

3.1.3 *United States of America*

Planning for seasonal influenza vaccination as well as pandemic vaccination was ongoing in the USA. The federal government was concerned that in the event of a pandemic, influenza vaccine manufactured outside the USA (accounting for about 40% of annual domestic seasonal supply) would be unavailable. Therefore, financial incentives were created during the past few years to help support the expansion and diversification of influenza vaccine manufacturing capacity in the USA. The desire to increase the amount of vaccine available in the USA was also pushed along by a recent ACIP recommendation to expand the use of seasonal vaccine to all those 6 months to 18 years of age. This age-based expanded recommendation helped to entice additional companies to make further long-term investments in their influenza vaccine program that included additional new and renovated influenza vaccine plants being built in the USA and elsewhere.

3.1.4 *Local Community/Wake Forest University Baptist Medical Center*

During the past decade, pandemic planning had occurred mostly at the federal and state level with much less planning in many of the local communities and at the individual level despite the fact that the actual implementation of the plan would need to occur at the local and individual level. Most of the pandemic planning in our community did not occur at the local government level, but at Wake Forest University Baptist Medical Center which is the academic medical center that serves as a regional referral center for western North Carolina. Disaster planning at Wake Forest University Baptist Medical Center had been ongoing for many years and pandemic planning for several years.

The ability to take the medical center's written plan and effectively implement it was now going to be tested and major concerns existed regarding how well this implementation would go. The anxiety initially proved well founded as implementation of the plan began in early May 2009. Problems occurred with sending communications to HCWs via email and other communication modalities about what to do with patients coming to the outpatient clinics and emergency department with influenza-like illness symptoms. These problems included corrupted email groupings, people with email boxes that were already full and those who don't read their emails on a regular basis. During this time the emergency department saw a substantial number of "worried well" patients who were afebrile with mild respiratory illnesses, although there had not yet been a confirmed case in North Carolina of infection due to the 2009 H1N1 virus. This would be a harbinger of what subsequently occurred when the second wave of the pandemic came through North Carolina and the outpatient and ICU surge capacities (i.e., the ability of medical centers to increase their ability to care for a large influx of additional patients in the outpatient and/or inpatient settings) were severely tested (surge capacity issues are discussed in Chapter 4).

Another problem that occurred at Wake Forest University Baptist Medical Center was that although the medical center initially had 68 courses of oseltamivir (each course contained enough medicine to treat one person), there was an immediate run on the outpatient pharmacy and within three hours there were only eight courses left. To ensure that there would be an adequate supply of oseltamivir to treat HCWs and patients going forward, this drug was put on the list of restricted antimicrobials which required that a form be filled out that noted the specific indications for its use, information that was reviewed by an infectious disease specialist. In conjunction with this requirement, additional courses of oseltamivir were purchased from the drug company (Roche). The hoarding of antiviral medications was not unusual as personal stockpiling of antiviral medications was reported to occur in >50% of medical centers across the USA.[36]

The 2009 H1N1 virus had started to spread throughout the USA in April and May 2009. The federal government decided to release some of the supplies from the Strategic National Stockpile to each state. In North Carolina, large numbers of regular masks and N95 respirators were shipped to a central location and then sent on to local communities (see Chapter 5 for an in-depth discussion of the controversy that developed over whether N95 respirators provided better protection than regular masks).

Soon thereafter, the first confirmed cases of 2009 H1N1 virus infection occurred in NC and this resulted in the NC Department of Public Health changing their recommendations for evaluation, testing and management of influenza-like illness so that:

- Regardless of travel/contact history, all patients who presented with influenza-like illness were now asked to put on a mask and placed in a separate room with the door closed (previously these restrictions were recommended only if the person with influenza-like illness had recently traveled to Mexico or California).
- Testing for 2009 H1N1 influenza would now only be performed on patients requiring admission to the hospital who presented with influenza-like illness without an alternate explanation.
- Testing for the 2009 H1N1 virus would no longer be performed on patients who presented with influenza-like illness but were not admitted to the hospital. Patients discharged from the outpatient setting were instructed to stay home until symptoms resolved, use hand, respiratory and cough hygiene, and call or seek emergency medical care, if warranted.
- Antiviral treatment with oseltamivir or zanamivir was now recommended only for patients requiring admission to the hospital or for those who were discharged from the outpatient setting with influenza-like illness and were at high risk for complications.
- All quarantine and isolation became voluntary for seven days and legal quarantine for those going home was discontinued.

Wake Forest University Baptist Medical Center had ordered 2,000 courses of oseltamivir ($81 per course) in April 2009, mainly to prevent and treat the disease in its HCWs, and in mid-May decided to purchase an additional 3,000 courses of this drug. This purchase was in addition to the oseltamivir that the state had shipped to local communities for use in people who developed influenza-like illness. Wake Forest University Baptist Medical Center also purchased 150 courses of Relenza as an alternative treatment for those who could not take oseltamivir by mouth. Additional antibacterial agents effective against *S. aureus* and *S. pneumoniae* were

45

purchased to treat secondary bacterial infections that were anticipated to occur as a complication of influenza.

Other planning issues that were initiated at Wake Forest University Baptist Medical Center involved developing a vaccine prioritization plan for HCWs with patient contact. This prioritization was considered necessary since it was unlikely that there would initially be enough vaccine available for all the HCWs at the medical center. Additionally, each clinical department was asked to develop inpatient and outpatient surge plans and submit them to the Pandemic Planning group to make sure that the various plans were not overlapping (e.g., to make sure that two clinical services were not planning to expand into the same inpatient or outpatient spaces). This planning proved helpful, but many adjustments to the plan were required as the first and second waves became more intense. Similar experiences were occurring in healthcare centers across the USA. A cross-sectional survey of members of the Society for Healthcare Epidemiology of America was done to evaluate the way in which healthcare institutions had responded to the first wave of the 2009 pandemic. Most centers indicated that they were reasonably well prepared to deal with the first wave, but identified further vaccine development and deployment, HCW education and revisions of pandemic influenza plans as important future initiatives.[36]

References

34. Human infection with new influenza A (H1N1) virus: Mexico, update, March–May 2009. *Wkly Epidemiol Rec* **84**: 213–219.
35. Smith GJ, Vijaykrishna D, Bahl J *et al.* (2009) Origins and evolutionary genomics of the 2009 swine-origin H1N1 influenza A epidemic. *Nature* **459**: 1122–1125.
36. Lautenbach E, Saint S, Henderson DK, Harris AD. (2010) Initial response of health care institutions to emergence of H1N1 influenza: Experiences, obstacles, and perceived future needs. *Clin Infect Dis* **50**: 523–527.

Chapter 4

The Pandemic is Declared: The First Wave Continues to Spread Globally (June through Mid-August 2009)

"The world is now at the start of the 2009 influenza pandemic, we are in the earliest days of the pandemic, the virus is spreading under a close and careful watch."

Dr. Margaret Chan, Director-General of the
World Health Organization, statement to the press announcing the
start of the 2009 influenza pandemic, June 11, 2009

4.1 A Pandemic is Declared: Phase 6 and the First Wave

4.1.1 *The Epidemiologic Features of the Pandemic Continue to Evolve*

A KEY POINT: The WHO officially declared the pandemic on June 11, 2009. Based on the previously established definition of phase 6 of a pandemic (i.e., an increased and sustained community spread of a new virus in the general population) the pandemic could have been declared weeks earlier. However, there were substantive social, economic and political reasons to hold off declaring this final phase until this time. These included the need for the WHO to hold a meeting where health ministers from all countries could receive information about the pandemic and give their input about what help they needed from the WHO. It was also important to prepare clear communications about the pandemic that would avoid unnecessary fear, while still motivating countries to increase the intensity of their pandemic planning.

4.1.1.1 *Worldwide*

On June 11, 2009, the WHO announced that the outbreak caused by the 2009 H1N1 virus was now in phase 6 and therefore the pandemic had gone from being imminent to officially declared. Less than nine weeks since the WHO first declared a public health event of international concern, and 41 years since the last influenza pandemic, there was now a new worldwide pandemic caused by a new virus that was a quadruple reassortant virus with genetic components from birds, pigs and humans. The rapid worldwide spread of disease is shown in Fig. 9 where the number of countries with laboratory-confirmed cases from early May compared to June 11, 2009, is depicted in two separate WHO maps.

In temperate countries, seasonal influenza virus can cause focal outbreaks in the summer, but overall there is minimal disease activity during this part of the year. This seasonal decrease in disease is thought to be due, in part, to the better viability of influenza viruses in the low humidity seen in the cooler months. However, during the summer of 2009, the 2009 H1N1 virus continued to cause disease throughout the Northern Hemisphere, especially in settings where there was prolonged close contact (e.g., summer camps). At the same time in the Southern Hemisphere, where the winter season had begun, the 2009 H1N1 virus initially co-circulated with other seasonal influenza viruses (Fig. 10), but soon became the predominant strain causing a high incidence of disease in many of these countries. The epidemiology and severity of the disease caused by the 2009 H1N1 virus in the Southern Hemisphere was reasonably similar to that seen in Mexico and the USA (Table 8).

During the first wave of the pandemic, the strain on the healthcare system was considerable, particularly in the ICUs. Worldwide estimates suggested that 1–10% of those who became ill due to the 2009 H1N1 virus were hospitalized and 10–25% of these patients required ICU care. A fatal outcome was recorded in 2–9% of hospitalized patients. Of all those hospitalized, 7–10% were pregnant women and they had a ~10-fold higher risk of requiring admission to the ICU when compared to the general population.

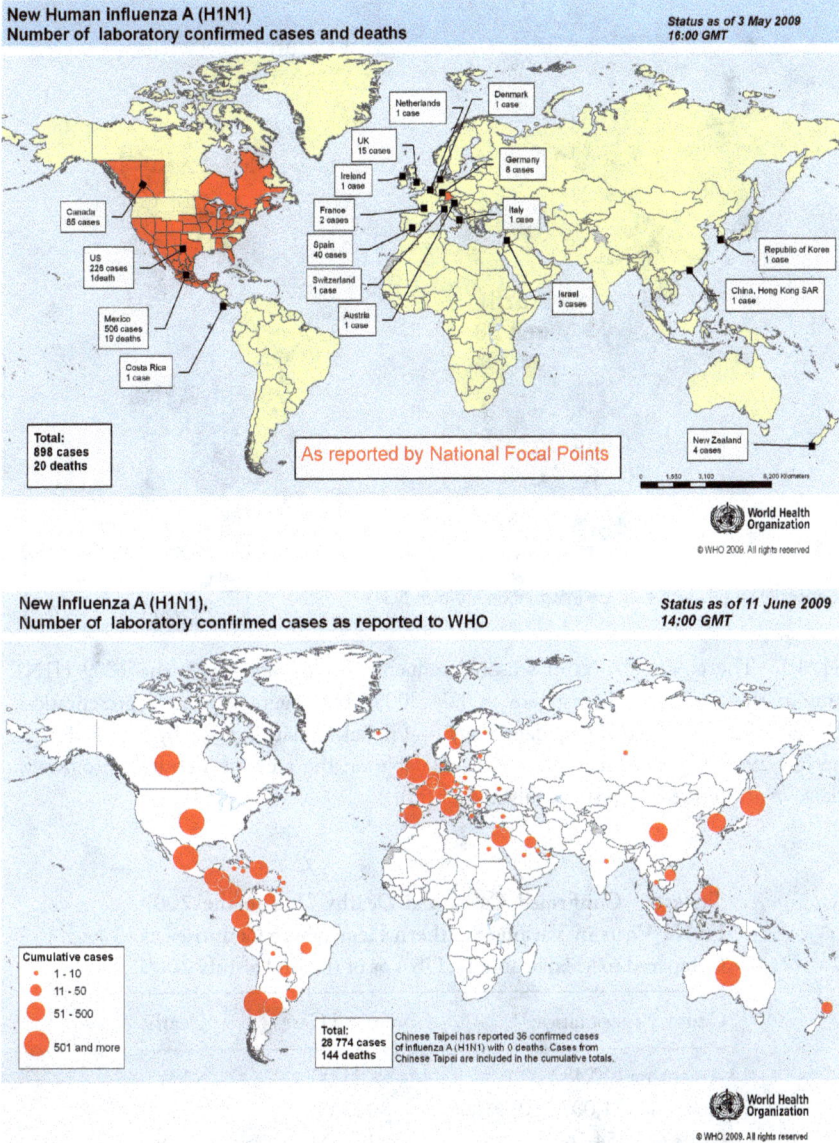

Fig. 9. The top WHO map was made available on May 3, 2009, and at that time there were 898 confirmed cases in 18 countries with 20 deaths. The bottom map is from June 11, 2009, when the WHO officially declared a pandemic (phase 6) and at that time there were 28,774 confirmed cases in 74 countries with 144 deaths. Data source: WHO Map Production: Public Health Information and Geographic Information Systems (GIS) (http://www.who.int/csr/disease/swineflu/updates/en/index.html).

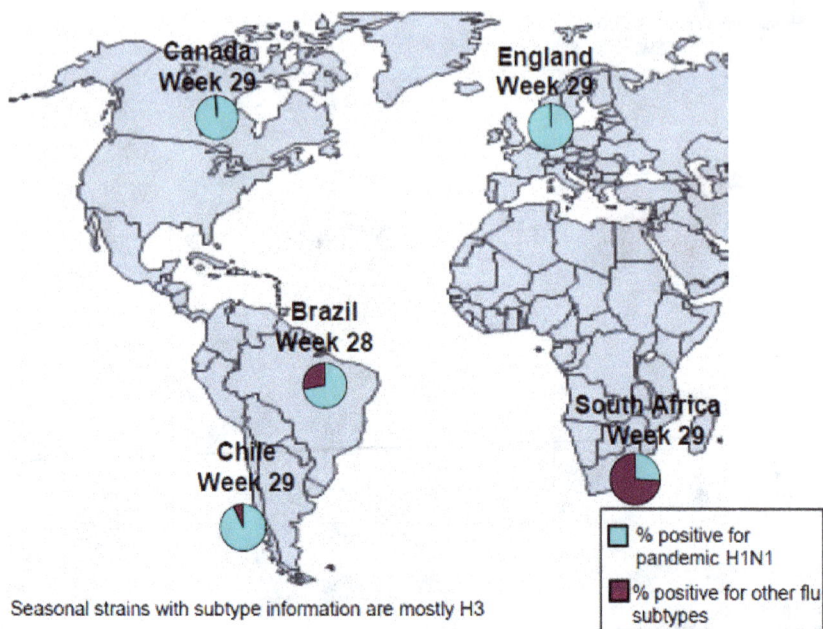

Fig. 10. The co-circulation of seasonal influenza strains along with the 2009 H1N1 virus in the Southern Hemisphere in July 2009. This figure is from a presentation, "Novel Influenza A(H1N1) Epidemiology — Global Update", given by Dr. J. Mott at the July 29, 2009 ACIP meeting and is available on the meeting website (http://www.cdc.gov/vaccines/recs/acip/slides-july09-flu.htm).

Table 8. Confirmed Cases and Deaths Due to the 2009 H1N1 Virus in Various Southern Hemisphere Countries as Compared to Mexico and the USA as of the End of July 2009

Country (population)*	Confirmed Cases	Deaths
Argentina (40,482,000)	>3,000	137
Australia (21,007,310)	>17,000	50
Chile (16,454,143)	>11,000	79
Mexico (109,955,400)	>12,000	124
USA (303,824,640)	>43,000	302

*The estimated population of each country as of July 2008.
The data were presented at the July 29, 2009 ACIP meeting.

In Australia and New Zealand, the overall ICU admission rate due to the 2009 H1N1 virus was ~29 per million people which was about 15 times greater than seen in previous influenza seasons.[37] The average age of those admitted to the ICU was 40 years and 68% of ICU patients had underlying risk factors including diabetes (16%), asthma or other chronic lung diseases (29%), chronic heart failure (11%), pregnancy (9%) and obesity (body mass index [BMI] >35 in 29%). Children <2 years of age and indigenous populations made up a much higher percentage of the population admitted to the ICU when compared to their prevalence in the general population. A Canadian study reported that intensive care capacity in Winnipeg, Manitoba, was "seriously challenged" at the peak of the outbreak with full occupancy of all regional ICU beds.[38] In certain areas of various countries (e.g., Argentina), patients had to be denied ICU care because of a shortage of available beds and/or personnel death (information presented at the Pan American Health Organization (PAHO) Immunization Meeting, Costa Rica, August 24–26, 2009).

4.1.1.2 *United States of America*

By the end of July, there were over 43,700 confirmed 2009 H1N1 cases in the USA and the CDC initial estimates suggested that there were greater than one million unconfirmed cases. The highest rate of confirmed illness occurred in patients 5–24 years of age (Fig. 11) with the median being ~12 years. The median age of hospitalized cases was 20 years (Fig. 12). There were over 5,000 hospitalizations and 300 deaths and the case fatality rate in confirmed cases was 0.7%. The age of those being hospitalized was substantially different from that in most influenza seasons as a greater percentage of those being hospitalized were school-age children, adolescents and adults <50 years of age rather than the elderly (Fig. 13). The greatest number of deaths occurred in young and middle-aged adults and the median age of fatal cases was ~37 years (Fig. 14). The majority of deaths during this first wave were caused by severe viral pneumonia that led to acute respiratory distress syndrome (ARDS) and this was different

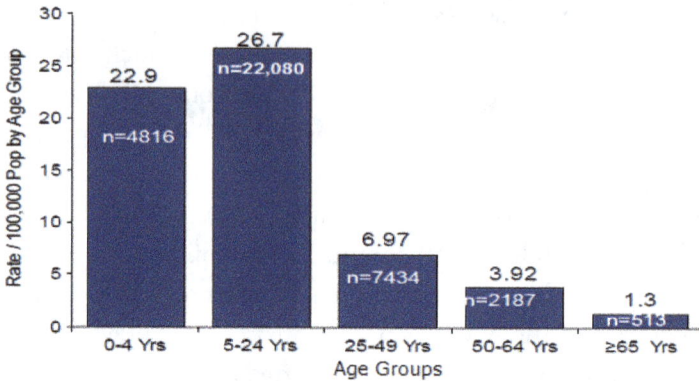

Fig. 11. The number (noted within the bar) and rate (noted on top of the bar) by age group of confirmed US cases due to the 2009 H1N1 virus. This figure is from a slide presentation, "Novel Influenza A(H1N1) Epidemiology in the U.S.", by Dr. Tony Fiore at the July 29, 2009 ACIP meeting (http://www.cdc.gov/vaccines/recs/acip/slides-july09-flu.htm).

from other epidemic and pandemic seasons where most deaths were due to secondary bacterial pneumonia.

Data from the CDC Emerging Infections Program obtained from April through August 2009 showed that 62% of those <18 years of age and 76% of adults who required hospitalization had underlying medical conditions. For those hospitalized, the incidence of co-morbidities was ≥50% in all age groups except those <2 years of age (Fig. 15). The most prevalent condition in hospitalized children and adults was asthma. Underlying medical conditions in children who died were mainly due to neurologic (52%), lung (38%) and cardiovascular (17%) diseases, while in adults the most common underlying conditions were due to lung (37%) and cardiovascular (26%) diseases as well as diabetes (24%). Morbid obesity (BMI > 40) was recognized as a possible risk factor for death for the first time. Table 9 compares the incidence of these and other underlying conditions for children and adolescents versus adults who were hospitalized or died.

The increased risk of hospitalization and death in pregnant women that occurred during the 2009 pandemic had also been noted in previous pandemics, especially in the 1918 pandemic where the reported mortality ranged from 27% to 45% and pregnancy loss was >50%.[39] While pregnant

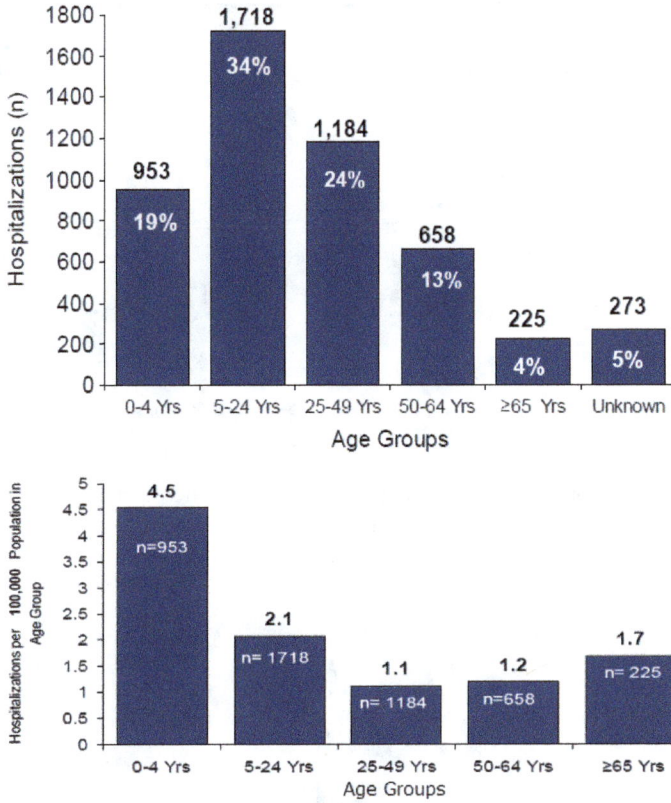

Fig. 12. The number (top figure) and rate (bottom figure) by age group of patients hospitalized in the USA due to the 2009 H1N1 virus. This figure is from a slide presentation, "Novel Influenza A(H1N1) Epidemiology in the U.S.", by Dr. Tony Fiore at the July 29, 2009 ACIP meeting (http://www.cdc.gov/vaccines/recs/acip/slides-july09-flu.htm).

women make up ~1% of the US population, they accounted for ~6% of the deaths that occurred in this first wave of the pandemic (Table 9). Many of these women did not have underlying chronic illnesses. Those pregnant women infected with the H1N1 virus that required hospitalization often developed rapid deterioration requiring prolonged ICU admission and mechanical ventilation due to primary viral pneumonia with subsequent ARDS. The risk of hospitalization and death increased over each trimester and extended into the first few weeks postpartum and also resulted in an increased incidence of premature births. The risk of this virus to

53

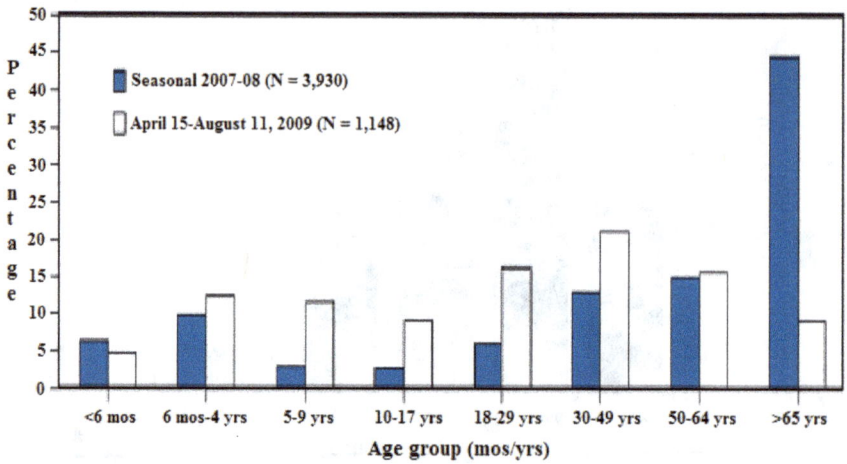

Fig. 13. A comparison of the distribution by age group of those hospitalized with laboratory-confirmed influenza in the USA during the 2007–2008 winter influenza season compared to the 2009 pandemic during the time period of April 15–August 11, 2009. *MMWR* (2009) **58**(early release): 1–8.

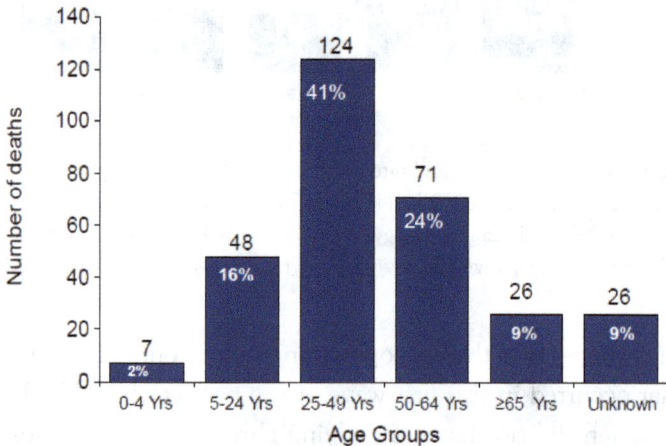

Fig. 14. The number of deaths in the USA by age group due to the 2009 H1N1 virus. This figure is from a slide presentation, "Novel Influenza A(H1N1) Epidemiology in the U.S.", by Dr. Tony Fiore at the July 29, 2009 ACIP meeting (http://www.cdc.gov/vaccines/recs/acip/slides-july09-flu.htm).

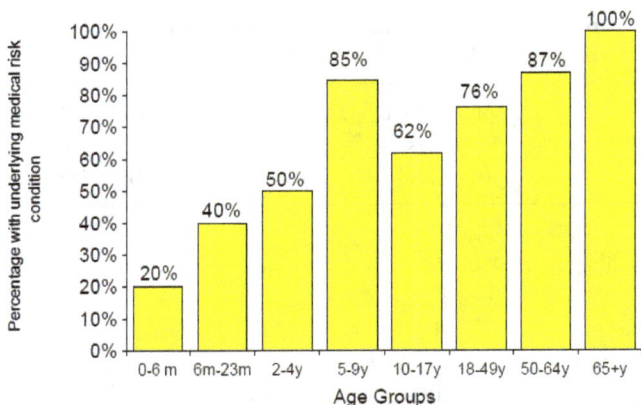

Fig. 15. The rate of co-morbidities that occurred in various age groups hospitalized due to 2009 H1N1 virus infection. This figure is from a slide presentation, "Novel Influenza A(H1N1) Epidemiology in the U.S.", by Dr. Tony Fiore at the July 29, 2009 ACIP meeting (http://www.cdc.gov/vaccines/recs/acip/slides-july09-flu.htm).

pregnant women was so concerning that in July 2009 British and Swiss health officials suggested that women in their countries should consider delaying pregnancy until the pandemic was over. This recommendation received substantial press coverage, but most other countries did not issue similar recommendations.[40]

The burden of this first wave of the pandemic on the healthcare system varied in different communities. In New York City, >2,500 patients per day visited outpatient facilities for influenza-like illness at the peak with 30–50 hospitalizations daily, while in some communities little disease was detected during the first wave. Further adding to the problem of caring for the increased number of people needing outpatient or inpatient care was that nosocomially and community-acquired 2009 H1N1 virus infections were occurring in HCWs. These events further increased the existing concerns about the need to increase surge capacity and prevent nosocomial transmission of the 2009 H1N1 virus to both HCWs and patients (see later in this chapter and Chapter 5 for additional surge planning that was done and the impact it had on these issues).

While the highest mortality rate during the first wave of the pandemic occurred in young and middle-aged adults, significant morbidity

55

Table 9. The Percentage of Pediatric and Adult Hospitalizations and Deaths Due to the 2009 H1N1 Virus by Underlying Medical Conditions*

Underlying Condition	Hospitalized (%)[+] ≤18 yrs (n = 465)	Hospitalized (%)[+] >18 yrs (n = 685)	Deaths (%)[¶] <18 yrs (n = 48)	Deaths (%)[¶] >18 yrs (n = 251)
Asthma	36	31	17	19
Other chronic lung disease	6	15	18	17
Cardiovascular	4	17	17	26
Neurologic diseases	11	6	52	12
Pregnancy	1	11	4	6
Diabetes	1	20	0	24
Renal	3	8	2	15
Cancer	—	4	6	16
Other immunosuppresive diseases	5	13	5	24
Hepatic and hematologic	7	—	2	17
Obesity	—	—	7	50

Adapted from a presentation at the October 23, 2009 ACIP meeting (http://www.cdc.gov/vaccines/recs/acip/slides-oct09.htm#fluvac).

*Some people had more than one underlying condition and therefore the numbers can exceed 100%.

[+]The CDC Emerging Infection Program survey included hospitalizations from April 15 to August 31, 2009, from those hospitals in the surveillance network.

[¶]The deaths were all those reported throughout the USA from April to June 2009.

— Estimate unreliable due to small sample size.

and mortality was also seen in children. From April through the first week in August, the CDC received reports of 477 deaths associated with the 2009 H1N1 virus in the USA, including 36 deaths in those ≤18 years of age. Seven (19%) of these children were <5 years of age, and 24 (67%) had one or more high-risk medical conditions. Twenty-two (92%) of the 24 children with high-risk medical conditions had neurodevelopmental conditions. Unlike the deaths that occurred in adults, the majority (63%) of the children who died had laboratory-confirmed bacterial co-infections.[41]

The WHO and CDC had stopped tracking the total number of pandemic cases by July 2009, since only a small proportion of persons with fever and respiratory illness were being tested and therefore the total number of confirmed cases was greatly underestimating the true incidence of disease. The CDC later estimated that during the first wave of the pandemic 1.8–5.7 million people had become ill in the USA due to the 2009 H1N1 virus and that 9,000–21,000 people had been hospitalized.[42] The CDC continued to collect and report weekly counts of pandemic H1N1-associated hospitalizations and deaths.

4.1.2 *Interventions Undertaken to Mitigate the Impact of the Pandemic*

> A KEY POINT: The WHO and CDC each issued revised vaccine prioritization schemes in July 2009 that were based on the current epidemiologic data and estimates of the amount of pandemic vaccine that would be available at various times over the next year. While there was little disagreement about what groups were at risk, there was a substantial difference between these two organizations regarding which groups would initially be recommended to receive the vaccine. The WHO prioritization scheme split at-risk populations into relatively small groups while the CDC lumped many at-risk populations together. These different recommendations were based on the relatively large percentage of the USA population the federal government anticipated it would be able to vaccinate by October 2009, compared to the much lower percentage of the population in developing countries the WHO believed would be vaccinated.

4.1.2.1 *Worldwide*

The Extraordinary Meeting of SAGE took place on July 7, 2009. The purpose of the meeting was to advise the WHO Director-General on the best way to mitigate the impact the pandemic on developing countries as the 2009 H1N1 virus vaccine became available. Additional participants in this meeting included non-SAGE members of the Ad Hoc Policy Advisory SAGE Working Group on Influenza A (H1N1) Vaccines, chairmen of the WHO regional technical advisory groups, partner organizations and external experts. Observers included industry representatives who did not take part in the recommendation process in order to avoid conflicts of interest. While the input from these non-SAGE representatives was important, the specific recommendations to the WHO Director-General came solely from the SAGE members. Specific questions considered at this meeting and their corresponding answers included:

(1) What was the worldwide production capacity to make a pandemic influenza vaccine and what was the time frame needed to make enough vaccine to fully implement a universal recommendation?

Worldwide there were >25 companies that made seasonal influenza vaccines, but the substantial majority of vaccine doses were made by seven of these companies (Table 10). Depending on information that would come

Table 10. Global Seasonal Trivalent Influenza Vaccine Production Capacity*

Companies	Total Annual Capacity (10^6 doses)	2008–2009 Northern Hemisphere Production (10^6 doses)	2009 Southern Hemisphere Production (10^6 doses)	2009–2010 Northern Hemisphere Production (10^6 doses)
Large companies[†]	560	300	103	323
Small companies[¶]	316	107	10	170
Total	877	470	113	493

*This table is from a slide presentation, "Update on A(H1N1) Pandemic and Seasonal Influenza Vaccine", by Dr. Marie-Paule Kieny at the WHO Extraordinary Strategic Advisory Group of Experts of Immunization meeting in Geneva, Switzerland, on July 7, 2009 (http://www.who.int/immunization/sage/previous_july2009/en).
[†]There are 7 vaccine companies that can each produce ≥2,000,000 doses of the 2009 pandemic vaccine.
[¶]There are 18 companies that can each produce <2,000,000 doses of the 2009 pandemic vaccine.

from animal and human studies during the next few months, it was possible that vaccine production could be further increased to as much as 93,000,000 doses per week which translated into ~5,000,000,000 doses in a year. Compared to even five years before, production capability was markedly increased due to a variety of factors including the decision in the USA to expand its influenza vaccination program to include all those from 6 months to 18 years of age and the expansion of annual influenza recommendations into 35 countries in Latin and South America. This recommendation increased the number of companies that decided to make influenza vaccines, while other manufacturers who were already making influenza vaccines substantially increased their production capacity. Additionally, the concern that the avian H5N1 virus might cause a pandemic led to the development of vaccines containing adjuvants. These adjuvants decreased the amount of viral protein needed to induce an immune response which in turn allowed for more doses of the pandemic vaccine to be produced (Table 11). The timeline for producing the 2009–2010 seasonal and pandemic vaccines worldwide is shown in Fig. 16.

Table 11. The Number of 2009 H1N1 Pandemic Vaccine Formulations Proposed by Various Manufacturers

	Whole	Split	Subunit	LAIV	Recombinant	Total
Number of vaccines of this type	9	14	4	5	1	33
Number of vaccines of this type which are adjuvanted	6	3	3	0	0	12

This table is from a slide presentation, "Update on A(H1N1) Pandemic and Seasonal Influenza Vaccine", by Dr. Marie-Paule Kieny at the WHO Extraordinary Strategic Advisory Group of Experts of Immunization meeting in Geneva, Switzerland, on July 7, 2009 (http://www.who.int/immunization/sage/previous_july2009/en).

(2) Should the manufacturing of the 2009–2010 Northern Hemisphere seasonal influenza vaccine be interrupted to allow for the start of production of a pandemic vaccine against the 2009 H1N1 virus?

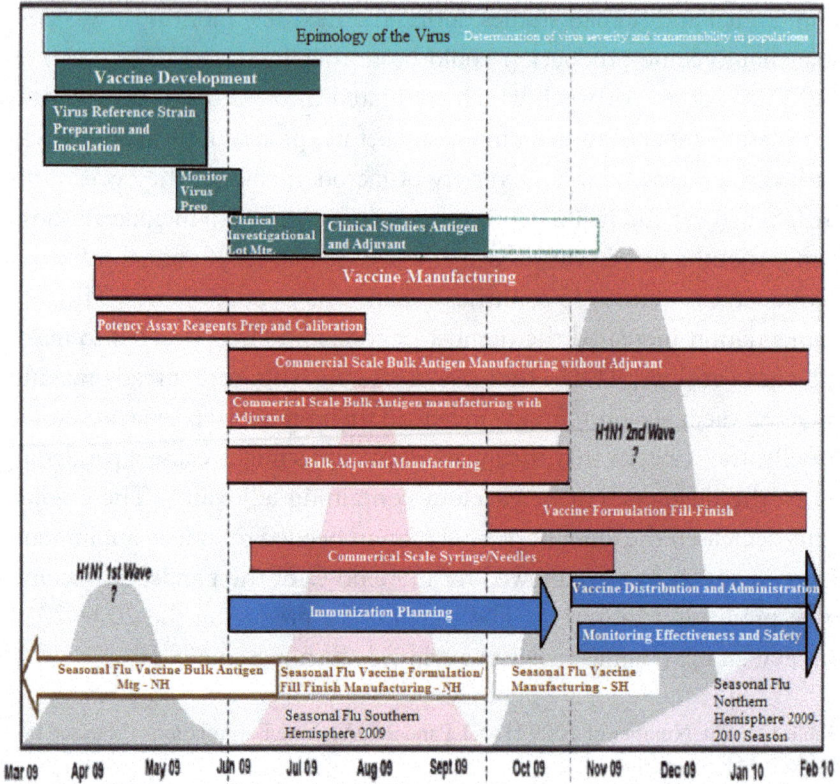

Fig. 16. A figure created by the United States Health and Human Services Biomedical Advanced Research and Development Authority (BARDA) to help as a planning tool. The figure shows a potential timeline for producing the 2009–2010 trivalent seasonal and monovalent pandemic influenza vaccines worldwide (https://www.medicalcountermeasures. gov/BARDA/documents/h1n1vacstrat508.pdf).

By this time of the July 7, 2009 meeting, the production of the 2009–2010 seasonal influenza vaccine in the Northern Hemisphere was almost complete. The total number of doses that the various companies had planned to make for the 2009–2010 season was 493,000,000 and by the end of July 2009, 92% of this total had already been made (Table 12). Therefore, SAGE felt that it was not necessary to recommend a "switch" from seasonal to pandemic vaccine production since the great majority of seasonal influenza vaccine had already been made and production would be

Table 12. The Status of Northern Hemisphere 2009–2010 Seasonal Vaccine Production by Date of Ascertainment

	Trivalent Seasonal Vaccine	
Date	Number of doses produced	% of total seasonal vaccine production
May 31, 2009	187,000,000	38
June 30, 2009	363,000,000	74
July 31, 2009	453,000,000*	92

*This is compared with the 470,000,000 doses produced during the 2008–2009 influenza season and the 493,000,000 total doses that were expected to be made for the 2009–2010 season.

This table is from a slide presentation, "Update on A(H1N1) Pandemic and Seasonal Influenza Vaccine", by Dr. Marie-Paule Kieny at the WHO Extraordinary SAGE meeting in Geneva, Switzerland, on July 7, 2009 (http://www.who.int/immunization/sage/previous_july2009/en).

completed before pandemic vaccine production could begin. SAGE did recommend that the production of the pandemic vaccine begin as soon as possible and the WHO advised that the pandemic vaccine would likely occur within the next few weeks.

While starting the production of the pandemic vaccine in July 2009 would not interfere with making the 2010–2011 seasonal vaccine in the Northern Hemisphere, which would not begin until February of 2010, there was concern that it might impact the availability of the 2010 seasonal vaccine made for the Southern Hemisphere whose production process would need to begin soon. The importance of this concern was highlighted by the epidemiologic data from the Southern Hemisphere where a significant amount of the disease occurring at the start of their 2009 winter season was due to a seasonal influenza virus in addition to the 2009 H1N1 pandemic virus (Fig. 10).

(3) If the decision was made to produce large quantities of the pandemic vaccine, what would be the deciding epidemiologic factors that should determine whether the vaccine should be used universally, selectively or not at all?

There was no doubt that the 2009 H1N1 virus was rapidly spreading across the world and data presented at the July SAGE meeting estimated the secondary attack rate to range from 19–43% in various countries.[43] Later, published studies reported even wider variability in attack rates from below 10% to as high as 61% and these figures were impacted by a number of factors including the age of those in the household (the older the age, the lower the attack rate and the use of antiviral prophylaxis.[44,45] The reproductive "R" number varied substantially in various communities with R values as low as 1.3 and as high as 3.3 as reported at the October 28, 2009 SAGE meeting (presentation by Simon Cauchemez and Neil Ferguson, http://www.who.int/immunization/sage/previous_october2009/en/index1. html) and in the literature.[31]

The attack rate and R value alone would not necessarily mean that the pandemic vaccine should be universally recommended. Another important issue was the severity of disease caused by this virus. The severity of the pandemic when taken from the perspective of an individual person is related to the virulence of the virus and the risk that the person will develop severe disease (i.e., do they have one or more risk factors that increase the risk of serious morbidity and mortality). The severity of the pandemic when taken from a population perspective is dependent on the virulence of the virus and the clinical attack rate. In the 2009 pandemic, the virulence of the virus was low for healthy individuals, but increased for those with high-risk conditions, and the attack rate varied substantially as noted above. Thus, SAGE was concerned that from a population perspective the impact of this pandemic would be substantial.[46] There were also concerns that as the 2009 H1N1 virus continued to circulate worldwide, it could undergo genetic mutations or reassortment with circulating human seasonal influenza or other animal viruses that might increase the virulence of the virus.

During the previous month, countries in the Southern Hemisphere had started to see a substantial increase in the number of cases as their winter season approached. Some of these countries had mortality rates similar to what the Northern Hemisphere had been experiencing, but in Argentina and some of the other countries in the Southern Hemisphere countries the mortality rates appeared to be substantially higher and their healthcare system was becoming overwhelmed. A report from Argentina indicated that the hospitalization rates for children were double those seen during the previous season with 19% of hospitalized children requiring care in the pediatric ICU. The estimated mortality rate was 1.1 per 100,000 children and this was 10 times greater than seen in the 2007 season.[47]

Even if the virulence of the 2009 H1N1 virus was similar to seasonal influenza, a high attack rate would mean that the number of people being hospitalized and dying would be greater than seen with seasonal influenza. Based on the information presented at the meeting, SAGE recommended maximum production of the pandemic vaccine.

(4) What safety, regulatory and programmatic issues need to be considered prior to a universal or selected use recommendation?

The major safety concern about using this vaccine related to the possibility that it might cause GBS. Various studies have examined whether seasonal influenza vaccine is associated with an increased risk of GBS with conflicting results regarding whether there is a small increased risk of GBS of 1–2 per million vaccine recipients.[48–50] Of particular concern was that a vaccine used widely in the USA in 1976 due to a local outbreak of a different H1N1 swine influenza virus in Fort Dix, New Jersey, was associated with GBS in approximately 1 per 100,000 vaccine recipients.[51] While the HA and NA proteins in the 1976 virus were substantially different from those in the 2009 H1N1 virus, the specific component of the 1976 swine influenza vaccine that may have caused GBS is unknown. Therefore, the concern about GBS remained and given the relatively rarity of GBS, this question could not be adequately answered prior to widespread use of the 2009 pandemic vaccine.

A further confounding issue related to whether the vaccine could cause GBS was that a number of studies have suggested that native seasonal influenza virus itself may be one of the causes of GBS.[49,50] SAGE therefore suggested that the WHO utilize the Global Polio Surveillance Network, that has been in place for many years to monitor the occurrence of polio virus-induced acute flaccid paralysis, as a way of studying the incidence of GBS due to the native 2009 H1N1 virus prior to the use of the pandemic vaccine. This surveillance could provide an estimate of the background incidence of GBS due to various inciting agents, including the 2009 H1N1 virus, prior to and after the use of the pandemic vaccine, and allow a determination of whether the pandemic vaccine can cause GBS.[52] The baseline rate of GBS in children <15 years of age was subsequently reported using data obtained from 2000 to 2008 from the acute flaccid surveillance system in Latin America and the Caribbean.[53] The average incidence of GBS was 0.8 cases per 100,000 children and differed significantly between northern and southern countries in this region.

A separate concern about the use of the pandemic vaccine was the very high likelihood that a decision to recommend universal vaccination would be associated with numerous side effects that would be spuriously linked to the vaccine because of temporal, rather than causative, associations. These spurious associations had occurred with every universally recommended vaccine and public concern tended to focus on selected long-term neurologic and autoimmune conditions (e.g., multiple sclerosis, rheumatoid arthritis, etc.). In the case of a pandemic vaccine that would be given on a mass scale this problem would be exacerbated. This problem made the need for a preplanned, clear communication strategy a high priority, in order that the public could be well informed about the difference between two events that are temporally associated versus two events where one causes the other.

Regulatory entities in various countries (e.g., the Food and Drug Administration) have their own requirements to license biologic products. Regulatory issues exist with any product that is developed, and when a product needs to be used in an emergency situation on a worldwide basis, these problems become even more acute and complex. Regulatory requirements vary to some extent between countries, but in emergency situations these agencies try to work together to harmonize requirements so that the process of bringing the vaccine to the worldwide market can be expedited. However, clinical trials are required and take time to complete, and in the case of the pandemic vaccine, they would be done in sequential age groups with healthy adults going before children and those with certain underlying conditions (e.g., HIV infection). The amount of data required by these regulatory agencies also varied and to a large extent depended on the perceived risk to benefit ratio that weighed the severity of the pandemic versus concerns regarding the safety and immunogenicity of the various vaccine formulations.

The European Medicines Agency had established a different approach from the USA Food and Drug Administration to the licensing of pandemic vaccines. The European Medicines Agency granted generalized approvals on the basis of "near relative" vaccines of what were anticipated to be potential pandemic viruses (e.g., H5N1) and then would grant a pandemic license as a strain change without requiring additional data once a pandemic virus occurred. This meant that a license could potentially be granted in a few days since they had already approved a related pandemic vaccine. The fact that GSK and Novartis already had approval for an H5N1 adjuvanted vaccine prior to the onset of 2009 H1N1 pandemic explains why adjuvanted vaccines were acceptable in Europe since the European Medicines Agency felt it had sufficient manufacturing and clinical data on adjuvanted vaccines while the Food and Drug Administration did not.

The WHO spent considerable time and effort to make sure that each regulatory entity would coordinate and streamline the information that would be required from the vaccine manufacturer to obtain a license to use the vaccine in various countries. One concern related to the fact that there were a large number of companies making different formulations of the vaccine (see Tables 10 and 11). A major issue involved the use of adjuvants in the vaccine. The potential advantages of adjuvants include the ability to use reduced amounts of viral protein to elicit an immune response, broader immunity against related strains of influenza virus and longer lasting immunity. The smaller the amount of protein needed, the greater the number of vaccine doses that can be made over a given period of time. The willingness of regulatory agencies to consider the use of an adjuvant was felt to be critical to the production of sufficient numbers of vaccine doses, particularly for use in developing countries.

Given that new formulations would be involved in the production of some pandemic vaccines, SAGE felt it was very important to implement post-marketing surveillance of the highest possible quality. Rapid sharing of the results of immunogenicity, post-marketing safety and effectiveness studies among the international community was essential for allowing countries to make necessary adjustments to their pandemic vaccination policies.

SAGE expressed concern that national regulatory decisions on the pandemic vaccines in developed countries could potentially adversely affect developing countries. Some of these decisions might reduce the global availability of vaccines. There could also be reluctance in developing countries to use a vaccine that had not been licensed in an industrialized country. SAGE encouraged countries to consider emergency provisions for use of unlicensed vaccines when contemplating potential vaccine use as part of their influenza preparedness plans.

Logistical issues would arise even if there were adequate quantities of the pandemic vaccine. Administering the vaccine to large numbers of people during a pandemic is fraught with a multitude of problems including the capacity to store large quantities of the vaccine, the associated supplies needed for their administration, transporting vaccine doses and other supplies to the sites where vaccination will occur, identifying sufficient numbers of personnel trained to administer the vaccine, and developing communications that adequately inform the public about the prioritization scheme and locations that will be used to administer the vaccine. These issues are further magnified in many developing countries where the infrastructure needed to deliver vaccines can be inadequate even in normal times.

(5) How should the pandemic vaccine be prioritized until a sufficient number of doses were available to immunize everyone for whom the vaccine was recommended?

SAGE identified three different objectives that countries could adopt as part of their pandemic vaccination strategy:

- protect the integrity of the healthcare system and the country's critical infrastructure;
- reduce morbidity and mortality; and
- reduce transmission of the pandemic virus within communities.

Since the spread of the pandemic virus was considered unstoppable, the vaccine was needed in all countries. SAGE emphasized the importance of striving to achieve equity among countries to access vaccines developed in response to the 2009 H1N1 virus pandemic. Given the relatively young demographic profile, the widespread prevalence of co-morbidities such as malnutrition, HIV/AIDS and tuberculosis, and the fact that some of these countries do not have well functioning healthcare systems, the 2009 pandemic could have a devastating impact on developing nations.

SAGE recommended that all countries should immunize their HCWs (1–2% of the global population) as a first priority to protect the essential health infrastructure. Since the quantity of vaccines initially available would not be sufficient to vaccinate everyone else, a step-wise approach to vaccinate particular groups should be considered. SAGE suggested the following groups for consideration, noting that countries might need to change the order of priority based on country-specific conditions: pregnant women (~2% of the world's population — an additional potential benefit of immunizing pregnant women was that recent studies suggested that vaccinating pregnant women would provide protection for their infants against influenza[54,55]); those aged above 6 months with high-risk chronic medical conditions; healthy young adults 15–49 years of age; healthy children; healthy adults 50–64 years of age; and healthy adults ≥65 years of age.

Countries could use a variety of vaccine deployment strategies to reach these objectives, but any strategy should reflect the country's epidemiological situation, resources and ability to access vaccines, to implement vaccination campaigns in the targeted groups, and to use other non-vaccine mitigation measures.

(6) Given that many of the developed countries had pre-existing contractual arrangements to buy pandemic vaccines from various vaccine companies, what steps could be taken to assure equitable distribution of the vaccine for people living in developing countries?

The WHO worked with the United Nations, various funding groups (e.g., Gates Foundation) and vaccine manufacturers to try to ensure that developing countries had access to the pandemic vaccine. Several companies

67

agreed to donate 10% of their vaccine supply to developing countries. Despite the vaccine donated by companies, by various developed countries and that bought by the United Nations, the issue of equitable distribution of the vaccine between high-, middle- and low-income countries remained a very big problem (Table 13), particularly when the size of the population is taken into account (Fig. 17).

SAGE emphasized the importance of striving to achieve equity among all countries wanting access to the pandemic vaccines and noted with great concern that in the current situation, a relatively small number of developed countries had access to most of the global vaccine output over the next 12 months through purchase agreements. SAGE commended the WHO for its efforts to collaborate with governments and industry to improve the timely access of low/middle-income countries to pandemic vaccines and to support the development of vaccine manufacturing capacity in developing countries.

The WHO Director-General endorsed the above recommendations a few days later, recognizing that they were well adapted to the current pandemic situation. She also noted that the recommendations would need to be changed if and when new epidemiologic data became available.

4.1.2.2 *United States of America*

At the ACIP meeting in June 2009, the USA Health and Human Services Biomedical Advanced Research and Development Authority (BARDA) announced that 40,000,000 doses of the pandemic vaccine should be available in the USA by October 2009, 120,000,000 doses of the vaccine by 2009, and 600,000,000 doses by March 2010 (enough to vaccinate everyone in the USA with two doses if needed). This represented a substantial increase from previous estimates and was based on the fact that during the past decade, the USA government had invested billions of dollars to increase the plant manufacturing capacity to make influenza vaccines and had contractual agreements to buy influenza vaccines from various companies with manufacturing plants inside and outside the USA. Based on these revised estimates of vaccine availability, the CDC announced

Table 13. Inequitable Distribution of the 2009 H1N1 Pandemic Vaccine Between High-Income and Low/Middle-Income Countries

Country Type*	Access Strategy	Population	Pandemic Vaccine Production Capacity as a % of the Total Population
High-income	Mostly open system — countries negotiate contracts with vaccine companies and some countries have vaccine manufacturing within their country	893,000,000	90
Low/Middle-income with capacity to make vaccine within the country	Mostly closed system — can manufacture some vaccine within their country. Limited or no plans to export vaccine to other countries	3,114,000,000	10
Low/Middle income with no capacity to make vaccine within the country	No current access to vaccines other than what WHO procures or companies donate	2,662,000,000	0

*High-income countries include the USA, Canada, Europe, Japan, Australia and others. Low/middle-income countries with local capacity to produce pandemic vaccine include Russia, China and India.

This table is from a slide presentation, "Update on A(H1N1) Pandemic and Seasonal Influenza Vaccine", by Dr. Marie-Paule Kieny at the WHO Extraordinary SAGE meeting in Geneva, Switzerland, on July 7, 2009 (http://www.who.int/immunization/sage/previous_july2009/en).

that there would be a specially called meeting of the ACIP on July 29, 2009, to determine if the USA vaccine prioritization scheme, which had been created in 2005 and last revised in 2008, would need to be changed.

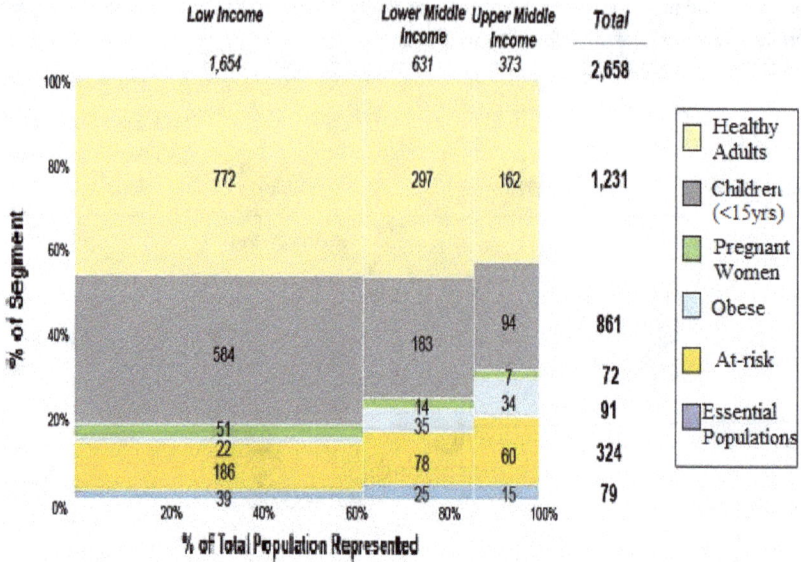

Fig. 17. Lack of equity between the distribution of the 2009 pandemic vaccine in high-income and low/middle-income countries determined when comparing the number of people with co-morbidities that make them at high risk for serious morbidity and mortality due to the 2009 H1N1 virus. The population numbers that are noted in the bar are in the millions. These data were presented at the WHO Extraordinary SAGE meeting in Geneva, Switzerland, on July 7, 2009 by Dr. Marie-Paule Kieny (http://www.who.int/immunization/sage/previous_july2009/en/).

At the June 2009 ACIP meeting, consideration was also given to using the polysaccharide pneumococcal 23-valent vaccine (PPV23) to help decrease the number of secondary bacterial infections due to S. pneumoniae during the 2009 pandemic. However, the epidemiologic data did not suggest that secondary pneumococcal infections were occurring at a high enough rate to warrant expansion of the current recommendations for that vaccine.

The ACIP met on July 29, 2009, and revised the 2008 vaccine prioritization scheme based on the following assumptions:

- The severity of illness and the groups at higher risk for infection or complications would be similar to what had initially been observed during the first wave.

- Antigen content, reactogenicity and immunogenicity of adjuvanted vaccine could not be assessed before trial data were available.
- The safety profile and antigen content of unadjuvanted 2009 pandemic vaccines would be similar to that of previous seasonal influenza vaccines.
- Enough vaccine doses for everyone in the USA would not be available before the likely occurrence of the second pandemic wave (presumed to be in the fall of 2009).
- The USA would have 120 million doses of pandemic vaccine ready for use by October 2009. Adequate supplies of licensed unadjuvanted vaccine could be produced for everyone in the USA by March of 2010.
- Two doses of pandemic vaccine would be needed to protect everyone.
- Pandemic vaccine and seasonal vaccine availability would overlap and both would be recommended for many populations groups.
- Initial demand for vaccination would be about the same as for seasonal vaccine, but could increase quickly if community transmission increases.
- Vaccine distribution would be timely, but there would still be mismatches between supply and demand at the local level.
- Implementation would pose many challenges.

The presumption that the amount of vaccine would be substantially greater than previously thought allowed many of the groups that were contained within tiers 1–4 in the 2008 scheme to now be included in the first priority tier (see Figs. 18 and 19 for the vaccine prioritization schemes done in 2008 and 2009, respectively). The criteria used to decide who would be placed in the top priority group were:

- Severity of illness and risk for complications due to the 2009 H1N1 virus.
- Likelihood of developing illness due to the 2009 H1N1 virus.
- Contribution to overall burden of severe illness.
- Protection of healthcare system functions.
- Reduction of societal impact.
- Potential for indirect protection of more vulnerable contacts.

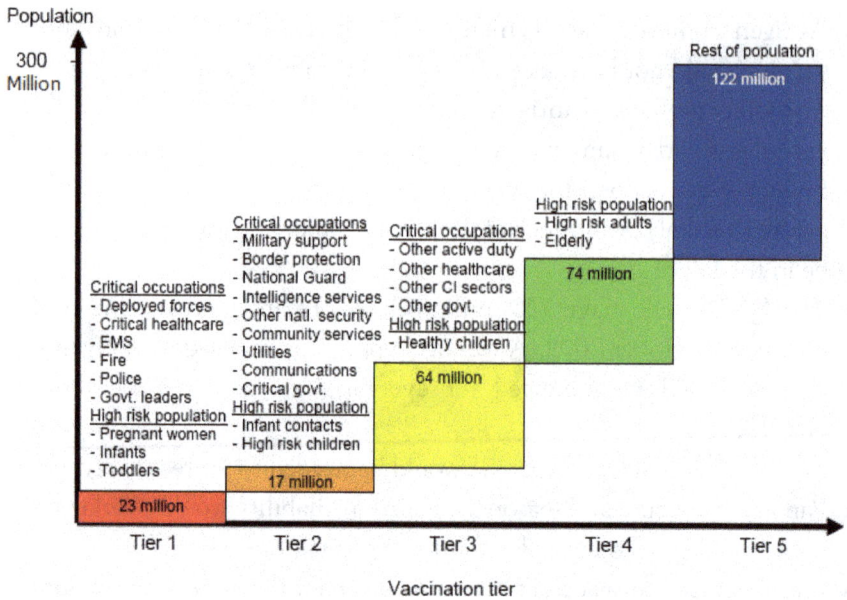

Fig. 18. The vaccination tiers and target groups for a severe pandemic published in 2008 and are a revision from the prioritization plan created in 2005. This figure illustrates how vaccination would be administered by tiers until the entire USA population had the opportunity to be vaccinated, and how tiers integrate target groups across the first four categories balancing vaccine allocation to occupationally defined groups and the general population.[56] Tier 1 includes the highest priority groups identified in each of the two categories (i.e., high-risk populations and critical occupations). Unlike other tiers which differ with severity of the pandemic, Tier 1 is the same across all pandemic severities. This tier is considered crucial for maintaining effectiveness of critical infrastructure or public sectors; burdens on these occupations are likely to be markedly increased in any pandemic, and risk of occupational exposure and infection is anticipated to be high due to contact with ill persons, living conditions or geographic locale. The report notes that the vaccine may be in extremely short supply through the first wave of a pandemic and it might be necessary to sub-prioritize vaccination of groups included in Tier 1 by stratifying within and between target groups.

Based on these parameters the following five groups, totaling 159 million people, were chosen to be in the first priority group:

(1) HCWs (~14 million people).

    a. Increased absenteeism would reduce healthcare system capacity and quality.

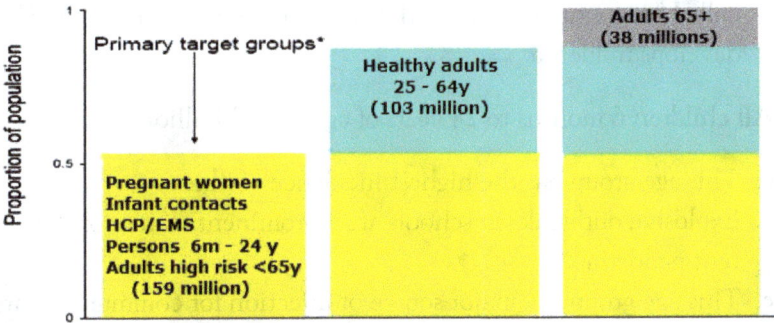

Fig. 19. The US vaccine prioritization plan as recommended by the ACIP during the July 29, 2009 meeting (http://www.cdc.gov/vaccines/recs/acip/slides-july09-flu.htm). The primary target group of 159 million people is based on the assumption that 120 million doses of pandemic vaccine would be available in the USA by October 2009. If less vaccine is available then a smaller subset of this group totaling 42 million people that includes pregnant women, contacts and care providers of infants <6 months of age, HCWs with direct contact with patients or potentially infectious material (e.g., microbiology laboratory technicians), children aged 6 months to 4 years and children 5–18 years with chronic medical conditions would get first priority for the vaccine.

b. The known occurrence of 2009 H1N1 virus infections among HCWs.

c. HCWs are a source of nosocomial infection for vulnerable patients.

(2) Pregnant women (~4 million women).

a. Higher risk of complications based on data from seasonal influenza, past pandemics and the current pandemic.

b. Potential for protection of infants <6 months of age who cannot be vaccinated, by preventing the mother from getting the disease and the possibility that passively transferred maternal antibodies could protect these infants.

(3) Household contacts and caregivers for children <6 months of age (~5 million people).

a. Young infants cannot be vaccinated.

b. Young infants are at higher risk for influenza-related complications and hospitalizations.

73

c. Immunizing everyone in the household to protect the infant is called "cocooning" and could decrease the chance that the infant develops influenza.

(4) All children 6 months to 24 years of age (~102 million people).

a. This age group has the highest incidence of illness.

b. Explosive outbreaks in schools are a prominent feature of the current pandemic.

c. This age group is a major source of infection for communities and in schools.

d. This age group has a higher incidence of hospitalizations compared to the older age groups.

e. Illness of children keeps parents at home.

(5) All adults 25–64 years of age with one or more co-morbidities including pulmonary, cardiovascular, renal, hepatic, cognitive, neurologic/neuromuscular, hematological or metabolic disorders, and immunosuppression (including immunosuppression caused by medications or by human immunodeficiency virus (~34 million people).

a. Approximately 70% of those hospitalized with 2009 H1N1 virus infections had a medical condition that confers higher risk for influenza-related complications.

The ACIP also considered a smaller first priority group if the amount of vaccine available by October 2009 was substantially less than was predicted. In this scenario, pregnant women, infant contacts, HCWs with direct patient contact, children 5–18 years of age with co-morbidities were included. All children 6 months to 4 years of age also remained in the highest priority group for a total of 42 million people. Healthy children 5–18 years of age, adults with co-morbidities, and HCWs with no patient contact were removed from the first priority group.

The difference between the WHO and CDC prioritization schemes relate mainly to the number of people who made it into the first priority group for vaccination. Both the WHO and CDC based their prioritization on the assumption that two doses of the pandemic influenza vaccine would be needed to immunize each individual. Given this assumption the WHO could only count on having enough vaccine to distribute to <10% of the population of developing countries by the end of 2009. In contrast, the USA prioritization scheme anticipated having 280 million doses of vaccine by the end of 2009 (120 million doses by October and then 80 million doses per month) which would likely be enough to vaccinate the first priority group with two doses of vaccine unless >85% of this group decided to get vaccinated. The federal government anticipated that there would be 600 million doses of vaccine by March 2010 which was enough to vaccinate everyone in the USA who wanted the vaccine.

However, on August 17, 2009, the government was forced to scale back the projected number of vaccine doses that would be available by October 2009 from 120 million to 45 million. This reduction was due to problems that vaccine manufacturers were having with the growth of the 2009 H1N1 virus in eggs which was 30% of what typically occurs with most strains of influenza virus used to make seasonal vaccine. Another problem with getting the vaccine out to the public was in developing the test needed to make sure doses are at the proper strength before they are cleared for use.

The CDC continued to develop new reference strains of the 2009 H1N1 virus that would have better growth characteristics, but it was clear that the amount of vaccine available by October would be substantially less than was projected in July 2009. Despite this lower projection, the CDC decided to let each local community decide if they would use the priority scheme that involved 159 million people or scale back to the prioritization plan for 45 million people. This flexibility was left in the program because the percentage of people in a given local community wishing to get vaccinated would likely vary widely and local public health officials could best decide if the demand for the vaccine was outstripping the amount of vaccine they had available.

4.1.3 *Consideration of Requiring Seasonal and Pandemic Influenza Vaccines for All HCWs*

> A KEY POINT: The issue of whether to make influenza vaccine mandatory in HCWs kept coming up during the past decade. The overall use of this vaccine in USA HCWs remained low (~45%) despite numerous educational efforts that highlighted the importance of this vaccine for the protection of HCWs and their families as well as patients. During the 2009 pandemic, a number of medical centers decided to mandate both the seasonal and pandemic vaccines for all HCWs.

By the end of July 2009 there had been 554 confirmed cases with 87 hospitalizations and 8 deaths in North Carolina. Pandemic planning at Wake Forest University Baptist Medical Center was continuing with increased intensity and strong consideration was being given to making the seasonal influenza and pandemic vaccines mandatory for all HCWs. The implementation of a mandatory influenza vaccine program had been contemplated for the past several years, but given that the influenza vaccination rate at Wake Forest University Baptist Medical Center had approached 80% during the 2007–2008 season, approximately two times the national average (Fig. 20), a mandatory policy had not been implemented. However, due to the potential impact of the 2009 pandemic on the Wake Forest University Baptist Medical Center workforce and its effect on the ability to care for patients this issue once again moved to the forefront.

Reasons in favor of implementing a mandatory influenza vaccine policy for HCWs included:

(1) Preliminary data obtained by the CDC suggested that 14% of HCWs likely became infected with the 2009 H1N1 virus from other HCWs.[57]
(2) HCWs have been infected with seasonal and the 2009 H1N1 influenza by patients and similarly patients have been infected by HCWs.[58–60]

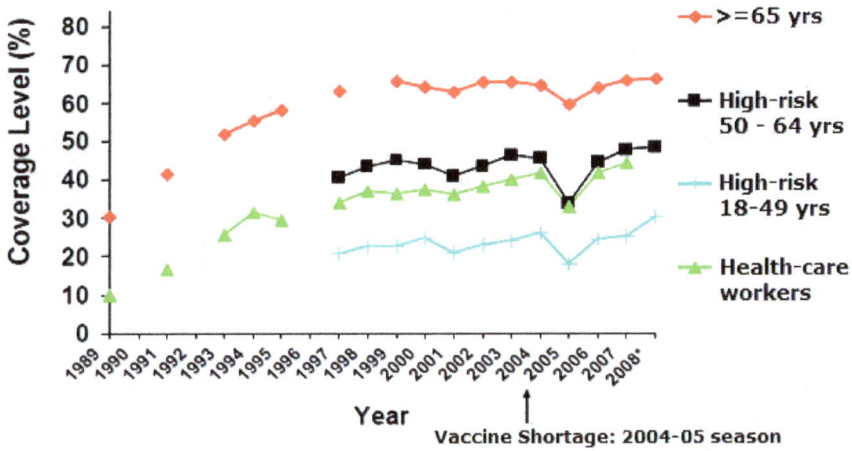

Fig. 20. Self-reported influenza vaccination coverage levels among selected high-priority USA adults in an ongoing national health interview survey. For 2008 the data is preliminary. This figure is from a slide presented at the July 29, 2009 ACIP meeting and is available on the meeting website (http://www.cdc.gov/vaccines/recs/acip/slides-july09-flu.htm).

(3) Vaccinating HCWs helps protect them from being infected in the medical or community setting and also reduces the chance they will infect patients they care for.

(4) HCWs that are out of work due to illness increase the number of patients that each HCW must care for and the resulting additional workload can result in decreased quality of care for patients.

(5) The highest incidence of hospitalization and death in the 2009 pandemic occurred in those 20–50 years of age. Most HCWs fall within this age range and many have co-morbidities that increase their risk of serious morbidity and mortality.

(6) Hospitals already mandate certain requirements for HCWs to protect themselves and their patients (e.g., rubella vaccination of employees who have negative rubella antibody tests). Thus, there is legal precedent for mandating vaccines for HCWs.

(7) Virginia Mason Medical Center in Seattle, Washington, was the first large healthcare organization to adopt a mandatory influenza vaccination policy in 2004. In 2008, Barnes-Jewish–Christian HealthCare

in St. Louis, Missouri, successfully established a mandatory influenza vaccine for their HCWs. Using this approach they vaccinated 98.4% of their 25,980 employees with 1.2% receiving medical exemptions (mainly for egg allergy or a history of GBS) and 0.3% religious exemptions. Eight employees (0.03%) who were not exempted refused vaccination and their employment was terminated.[61] Other large healthcare organizations and academic medical centers, including Hospital Corporation of America, Johns Hopkins Health System, University of Iowa Hospitals and the University of Pennsylvania Children's Hospital, had indicated they were in the process of initiating a mandatory influenza vaccination program for the 2009–2010 season.[58] Additionally, the New York State Department of Health announced on August 13, 2009, that influenza vaccination would now be a requirement for all hospital staff in New York State as a condition of employment, but the legality of a statewide policy was subsequently challenged in court and a temporary restraining order was issued until three lawsuits could be tested in court.[62]

(8) Several hospitals in North Carolina had already experienced substantial disruption in their clinical operations because of nosocomial infections due to the 2009 H1N1 virus in their neonatal intensive care and transplant units.

Reasons against implementing a mandatory vaccine policy for HCWs included:

(1) There were many logistical issues that had to be overcome to vaccinate every HCW at the medical center. The 2009–2010 influenza campaign required one dose of the seasonal vaccine and potentially two separate doses of the pandemic vaccine. The seasonal vaccine started to become available for use in August 2009. The pandemic vaccine would not be expected to become available until October 2009 and if a two-dose regimen was needed the doses had to be given at least three weeks apart. Additionally, the pandemic vaccine would likely not be available in sufficient amounts to immunize all

the HCWs at Wake Forest University Baptist Medical Center at the same time, and therefore a prioritization scheme needed to be created.

(2) There was an increased cost for mandating the seasonal and pandemic vaccine. For the seasonal vaccine, there was the cost of buying and administrating the extra vaccine doses that were needed (the influenza vaccination rate at Wake Forest University Baptist Medical Center for the 2008–2009 season was 75% and under a mandatory policy would approach 100%, since only a small number of HCWs had contraindications that would exempt them from getting vaccinated). The pandemic vaccine and supplies would be paid for by the federal government, but the increased personnel and other costs needed to vaccinate everyone would not be reimbursed. Overall, the estimated increase in cost was ~$60,000.

(3) The question of whether the pandemic vaccine would cause GBS was a major safety concern because of the previously discussed events that occurred in 1976 when the use of an influenza vaccine was associated with GBS in ~1 per 100,000 people vaccinated. This rate was a ~10-fold increase over the background GBS incidence seen in other seasonal influenza vaccine campaigns. While no one could say with absolute certainty that the 2009 novel influenza vaccine would not be associated with an increased rate of GBS cases, the circumstances in 1976 and 2009 were very different. The biggest difference was that the 1976 swine flu outbreak involved ~200 soldiers at Fort Dix, New Jersey, and never spread outside this army base. The 2009 H1N1 virus was clearly causing a worldwide pandemic with many millions of cases in the USA and elsewhere. Thus, the risk/benefit analysis concerning whether and how to use the 2009 pandemic vaccine was very different.

(4) Worldwide, different formulations of pandemic vaccine (e.g., adjuvants, recombinant antigens, etc.) were being made for use in the 2009 pandemic and many of these formulations had not been used in previous years. However, only unadjuvanted vaccine was designated

for use in the USA and this vaccine was the same formulation that had been used for decades. Thus, for USA HCWs, this issue was not really relevant, but many HCWs remained concerned that this was an "untested vaccine" despite being informed that it was being made by the same process used for many decades to make seasonal influenza vaccines.

4.1.4 *Antiviral Treatment and Prophylaxis Issues*

A KEY POINT: During the past decade, the emergence of resistance of H3N2 seasonal influenza viruses to the adamantane drugs and H1N1 seasonal viruses to the neuraminidase inhibitor drugs made it clear that reliance on antiviral drugs as the major weapon in treating and preventing infections during a pandemic was fraught with hazard. At the onset of the current pandemic, the 2009 H1N1 virus was resistant to the adamantanes and resistance to the neuraminidase inhibitors soon started to occur in a small number of virus isolates. This led the CDC to further narrow the treatment and prophylaxis indications for the use of the neuraminidase inhibitors.

As part of the worldwide pandemic planning process, ~220 million treatment courses of oseltamivir (ten capsules taken over five days) had been sold by Roche Pharmaceuticals to a large number of countries since 2000. Some of these courses had been used to treat seasonal influenza, but most remained in the stockpiles until the onset of the current pandemic. Roche licensed several other producers to make a generic version of the drug and this was estimated to increase the amount of oseltamivir that could be made to ~400 million courses per year. Additionally, in August 2009, regulatory agencies in many countries increased the shelf life of oseltamivir from five to seven years and this extension meant that the existing drug stockpiles whose expiration date was approaching could now be used during the 2009 pandemic. However, the WHO estimated that up to two billion people could become infected with the 2009 H1N1 virus, making it clear that this drug could not be used to treat everyone.

Initially, oseltamivir was widely prescribed for both treatment and prophylaxis of the 2009 H1N1 virus, but the CDC soon began to issue recommendations about the use of oseltamivir and zanamivir that were more restrictive as epidemiologic data about who was at risk for serious morbidity and mortality became available and concerns about the development of resistance of the 2009 H1N1 virus started to increase. Additionally, for most otherwise healthy people the impact of the treatment on the course of their disease appeared to be modest.

The initial recommendations included treatment with a neuraminidase inhibitor (oseltamivir or zanamivir) of hospitalized patients known to be at higher risk for seasonal influenza since at that point there was very little known about the specific risk factors for severe outcome due to the 2009 H1N1 virus. Those recommended for treatment included hospitalized patients >65 or <5 years of age or those with certain underlying medical conditions. Post-exposure prophylaxis with these same drugs was recommended for these high-risk groups if they had exposure to a confirmed case. HCWs were also to receive prophylaxis if they were not using appropriate protective equipment during close contact with a confirmed, probable or suspect case of 2009 H1N1 infection during the time the patient was considered infectious.

During the summer of 2009, most of the circulating 2009 H1N1 viruses remained susceptible to oseltamivir and zanamivir, but resistant to amantadine and rimantadine. A small number of patients with oseltamivir-resistant H1N1 virus infections were reported, but these cases were not in contact with each other and therefore there was no heightened concern that these oseltamivir-resistant virus isolates were being transmitted person-to-person. However, in August 2009, the CDC reported oseltamivir resistance in 2009 H1N1 virus isolates from two epidemiologically linked patients in North Carolina. Both developed illness in July while receiving oseltamivir chemoprophylaxis which was used widely in those attending a summer camp, after a presumed exposure to an ill person in the camp. Their illnesses were mild and resolved without complications. While there was no evidence of ongoing transmission of oseltamivir-resistant 2009 H1N1 virus, the North Carolina Health Department re-emphasized the following recommendation about the use of these antiviral agents:

- Antiviral chemoprophylaxis should be used judiciously to decrease opportunities for development of antiviral resistance.
- Chemoprophylaxis for prevention of illness in healthy children or adults following exposure to ill persons is not indicated.
- Antiviral chemoprophylaxis may be considered for persons at higher risk for complications due to influenza or for some HCWs with an exposure to the 2009 H1N1 virus secondary to inadequate personal protective equipment use.
- Careful observation for symptoms following an exposure, combined with early treatment if symptoms develop, could be an appropriate alternative to chemoprophylaxis in some settings, and could reduce the potential for oseltamivir resistance.
- Development of symptoms while receiving prophylaxis does not necessarily indicate antiviral resistance.
- Healthy patients with uncomplicated illness need not be treated with antivirals.
- Antiviral treatment with either oseltamivir or zanamivir is recommended for all patients with confirmed, probable or suspected cases of 2009 H1N1 virus infection who are hospitalized or who are at higher risk for influenza complications.
- If antiviral treatment is indicated in a patient whose symptoms developed >48 hours after beginning oseltamivir prophylaxis, consider use of zanamivir if the patient is ≥7 years of age and does not have underlying airway disease.
- Isolation of ill persons, good hand and respiratory hygiene, and vaccination (when available) should be the cornerstones of strategies to prevent transmission of the 2009 H1N1 virus.

4.1.5 *Communication Issues*

A KEY POINT: A multitude of communication issues arose from the decision to recommend the use of the pandemic vaccine. The most difficult one was striking the right balance between informing the public about the seriousness of the pandemic and the need to be vaccinated while at the same time not causing a panic. Public health authorities were concerned that a substantial percentage of the population would continue to think of influenza as a "bad cold", while others would be very upset if they were not included in the highest priority group to get the vaccine when it first became available.

During the past decade, the CDC and other organizations had conducted large-scale education campaigns about the seriousness of seasonal influenza and the ability of influenza vaccine to protect against this disease. Despite the fact that influenza is the leading cause of vaccine-preventable disease in the USA, these educational efforts have not resulted in the CDC reaching its Healthy People 2010 goal that 60% of high-risk adults should be vaccinated against influenza (Fig. 20).[63]

The combination of sound science being used to create a pandemic prevention and a treatment policy with effective communication about the rationale for the policy can save lives by increasing the number of people who get vaccinated and receive timely treatment if they become ill. Striking the right balance between making sure the public understands the importance of being vaccinated against both seasonal and pandemic influenza and not scaring the public is a difficult task. Dr. Joseph Bresee, Chief of the CDC Influenza Epidemiology and Prevention Branch, addressed this issue when he stated that "Hopefully, we will not have a panic, but instead we will have the appropriate level of concern and response."[64]

Research done by the CDC during the first wave of the pandemic indicated that a high percentage of the USA population was aware of seasonal and pandemic influenza, but a minority of people perceived the seasonal or 2009 H1N1 virus to be a serious threat to themselves or their families. As the first wave of the pandemic progressed, there was a relatively low desire to get the vaccine due to the perception of a low threat from the disease, safety concerns about a new pandemic vaccine and the likely need for two doses. A Gallup poll done after the WHO declared the pandemic on June 11, 2009, indicated that only 8% said they worried about getting sick from the 2009 H1N1 virus which was down from 25% when a similar survey was done after the initial outbreak in April 2009.

Other major communication problems included the need for public health authorities to frequently adjust their various recommendations based on the evolving epidemiology of the pandemic. The changing recommendations were based on new data about specific risk factors for developing severe disease (e.g., pregnancy, obesity, etc.) and what interventions might be effective in preventing and treating disease. Initially the CDC recommended school closings if a single case occurred in a school, but due to the low proportion of severe cases in otherwise healthy individuals this recommendation was soon changed. These frequently changing messages were confusing for the public. Further adding to the confusion was a variety of disparate messages in the lay press and on internet sites. While a great deal of time, effort and resources were committed to develop clear and concise messages, these efforts were only partially effective in maximizing the impact of the public health advisories.

4.1.6 *Concern that the Pandemic's Second Wave Would Soon Begin*

A KEY POINT: The history of pandemics indicates that a second wave frequently follows the first wave and its impact is usually more severe. The WHO and CDC were concerned that the peak of the second wave in the Northern Hemisphere would occur in the early fall prior to the time that the pandemic vaccine would be available in sufficient quantities for use in the first priority group, no less the entire population.

4.1.6.1 *Worldwide*

During the first wave of the pandemic substantially more people were infected with the 2009 H1N1 virus than the actual number of cases that were confirmed in various countries. However, only a minority of the population in each country had been infected, and therefore the majority of people were still susceptible to infection with the 2009 H1N1 virus during a second wave. During the last week of August, the WHO issued a briefing note "Preparing for the Second Wave: Lessons from Current Outbreaks". The basis for this report was the epidemiologic data coming in from the Southern Hemisphere and the knowledge that large numbers of people in all countries remained susceptible to infection. Even if the current pattern of usually mild illness continued in otherwise healthy people, the impact of the pandemic during the second wave would likely worsen as a greater percentage of the population became infected. Larger numbers of severely ill patients requiring intensive care would place a greater burden on health services, creating pressures that could overwhelm ICUs and also interfere with the provision of care for people with other diseases.

The WHO noted that during the winter season in the Southern Hemisphere, a number of countries had viewed the need for intensive care as the greatest burden on health services. Some cities in these countries reported that >15% of hospitalized cases required intensive care. The WHO warned that preparedness measures need to anticipate this increased demand on ICUs, which could be overwhelmed by a sudden surge in the number of severe cases.

The WHO warned that health officials need to be aware that many of the conditions that predispose people to severe disease had become much more widespread in recent decades, thus increasing the pool of vulnerable people. The WHO estimated that, worldwide, more than 230 million people suffer from asthma, and more than 220 million people have diabetes. Obesity, which was present in many severe and fatal cases of 2009 H1N1 virus infection, is now a global epidemic. Additionally, several preliminary studies showed a higher risk of hospitalization and death among certain population subgroups, including minority groups and indigenous populations. Early deaths from such conditions, precipitated by infection with the H1N1 virus, were another dimension of the pandemic's impact.

4.1.6.2 *United States of America*

Around the same time, the President's Council of Advisors on Science and Technology issued the "Report to the President on U.S. Preparations for 2009 H1N1 Influenza". The members of this group appointed by President Obama, included a number of highly respected scientists whose job was to advise the President on a wide range of scientific issues. This report provided recommendations to help guide the response to the anticipated second wave of the pandemic. The report assessed the likely scale of this second wave and the capacity of the USA to respond to it. The group indicated that they believed the most plausible scenario would be that "By the end of 2009, 60 to 120 million Americans would have experienced symptomatic infection with 2009–H1N1; nearly 1 to 2 million would have been hospitalized, with about 150,000–300,000 cared for in ICUs; and somewhere between 30,000 and 90,000 people would have died, the majority of them under 50 years of age" (www.ostp.gov/cs/pcast).

The President's Council of Advisors on Science and Technology was favorably impressed with the federal pandemic response including the wide range of issues that had been anticipated and addressed and the awareness of potential problems that would likely still occur even though they had been considered. The two main planning areas that were felt to need further refinement were vaccine production and surge capacity in the ICUs. The main problem with the pandemic vaccine was that the first significant quantities of vaccine were predicted not to be available until the middle of October 2009 and once a person was vaccinated it would take approximately two weeks to develop an immune response if only one dose was needed and longer if two doses were required. If the prediction that the resurgence of the epidemic would start in September and peak in mid-October was correct, then a vaccination campaign would not begin to protect vaccinees until well after the second wave had peaked (this issue is discussed in greater detail in Chapter 5). Their report noted that in the USA, the ICU occupancy level normally runs at ~80% of capacity and that during the 2009 pandemic people requiring ICU care, including those needing mechanical ventilation, could run as high as 25 per 100,000 population. If true, this would exceed the total ICU capacity in the USA by more than 100%. These estimates were within the range generated by other modelers. A summary and bibliography for these estimates can be found at: "Mortality and Morbidity Burden Associated with A/H1N1pdm Influenza Virus" (http://knol.google.com/k/markmiller/mortalityandmorbidityburden/1y43 omtho1mv6/3?collectionId=28qm4w0q65e4w.1&position=1#).

The President's Council of Advisors on Science and Technology report highlighted several other important issues that could directly impact the ability to care for increased numbers of patients in ICUs. The adequacy of supplies, particularly ventilators, might limit the number of patients that could be cared for in the ICU setting. Concern was noted about the number of available pediatric intensive care units (PICUs), since many community hospitals do not have PICUs and do not have trained personnel capable of caring for children in adult ICUs. The lack of adequate numbers of ICU-trained personnel able to care for adult and pediatric patients might be further exacerbated given that many HCWs could be out due to illness caused by the 2009 H1N1 virus. HCWs being out due to illness could be particularly problematic until the initial lots of vaccine were available to immunize the first priority group which includes HCWs. Furthermore, the problem could continue even after the first priority group was immunized, since some HCWs who were not themselves ill would likely stay at home to take care of sick family members. Embedded in this issue is the question of how many HCWs (and their family members) would agree to get vaccinated.

The WHO and President's Council of Advisors on Science and Technology reports made one thing clear: The second wave was likely to occur and we would soon find out what the true impact would be.

References

37. ANZIC Influenza Investigators, Webb SA, Pettilä V, Seppelt I *et al.* (2009) Critical care services and 2009 H1N1 influenza in Australia and New Zealand. *N Engl J Med* **361**: 1925–1934.
38. Kumar A, Zarychanski R, Pinto R *et al.*; Canadian Critical Care Trials Group H1N1 Collaborative. (2009) Critically ill patients with 2009 influenza A (H1N1) infection in Canada. *JAMA* **302**: 1872–9.
39. Rasmussen SA, Jamieson DJ, Bresee JS. (2008) Pandemic influenza and pregnant women. *Emerg Infect Dis* **14**: 95–100.
40. Stobbe M. (2009) Pregnant women may be among first to get swine flu shots; they account for 6 percent of deaths. *The Associated Press.*
41. Centers for Disease Control and Prevention (CDC). (2009) Surveillance for pediatric deaths associated with 2009 pandemic influenza A (H1N1) virus infection – United States, April–August 2009. *MMWR* **58**: 941–947.
42. Reed C, Angulo FJ, Swerdlow DL *et al.* (2009) Estimates of the prevalence of pandemic (H1N1) 2009, United States, April–July 2009. *Emerg Infect Dis* **15**: 2004–2007.
43. WHO Extraordinary Strategic Advisory Group of Experts on Immunization meeting, July 7, 2009 [http://www.who.int/immunization/sage/previous_july2009/ en/].
44. France AM, Jackson M, Schrag S *et al.* (2010) Household transmission of 2009 influenza A (H1N1) virus after a school-based outbreak in New York City, April–May 2009. *J Infect Dis* **201**: 984–992.
45. Fraser C, Donnelly CA, Cauchemez S *et al.* (2009) Pandemic potential of a strain of influenza A (H1N1): Early findings. *Science* **324**: 1557–1561.
46. Mathematical modelling of the pandemic H1N1 2009. (2009) *Wkly Epidemiol Rec* **84**: 341–348.
47. Libster R, Bugna J, Coviello S *et al.* (2010) Pediatric hospitalizations associated with 2009 pandemic influenza A (H1N1) in Argentina. *N Engl J Med* **362**: 45–55.
48. Lasky T, Terracciano GJ, Magder L *et al.* (1998) The Guillain-Barré syndrome and the 1992–1993 and 1993–1994 influenza vaccines. *N Engl J Med* **339**: 1797–1802.
49. Sivadon-Tardy V, Orlikowski D, Porcher R *et al.* (2009) Guillain-Barré syndrome and influenza virus infection. *Clin Infect Dis* **48**: 48–56.

50. Stowe J, Andrews N, Wise L, Miller E. (2009) Investigation of the temporal association of Guillain-Barre syndrome with influenza vaccine and influenza-like illness using the United Kingdom General Practice Research Database. *Am J Epidemiol* **169**: 382–388.

51. Schonberger LB, Bregman DJ, Sullivan-Bolyai JZ *et al.* (1979) Guillain-Barre syndrome following vaccination in the National Influenza Immunization Program, United States, 1976–1977. *Am J Epidemiol* **110**: 105–123.

52. Evans D, Cauchemez S, Hayden FG. (2009) "Prepandemic" immunization for novel influenza viruses, "swine flu" vaccine, Guillain-Barré syndrome, and the detection of rare severe adverse events. *J Infect Dis* **200**: 321–328.

53. Landaverde JM, Danovaro-Holliday MC, Trumbo SP *et al.* (2010) Guillain-Barré syndrome in children aged <15 years in Latin America and the Caribbean: Baseline rates in the context of the influenza A (H1N1) pandemic. *J Infect Dis* **201**: 746–750.

54. Zaman K, Roy E, Arifeen SE *et al.* (2008) Effectiveness of maternal influenza immunization in mothers and infants. *N Engl J Med* **359**: 1555–1564.

55. France EK, Smith-Ray R, McClure D *et al.* (2006) Impact of maternal influenza vaccination during pregnancy on the incidence of acute respiratory illness visits among infants. *Arch Pediatr Adolesc Med* **160**: 1277–1283.

56. US Department of Health & Human Services. Draft Guidance on Allocating and Targeting Pandemic Influenza Vaccine [http://www.pandemicflu.gov/vaccine/prioritization.html].

57. Srinivasan A, Perl TM. (2009) Respiratory protection against influenza. *JAMA* **302**: 1903–1904.

58. Pavia AT. (2010) Mandate to protect patients from health care-associated influenza. *Clin Infect Dis* **50**: 465–467.

59. Cunney RJ, Bialachowski A, Thornley D *et al.* (2000) An outbreak of influenza A in a neonatal intensive care unit. *Infect Control Hosp Epidemiol* **21**: 449–454.

60. Salgado CD, Farr BM, Hall KK, Hayden FG. (2002) Influenza in the acute hospital setting. *Lancet Infect Dis* **2**: 145–155.

61. Babcock HM, Gemeinhart N, Jones M *et al.* (2010) Mandatory influenza vaccination of health care workers: translating policy to practice. *Clin Infect Dis* **50**: 459–464.

62. Hartcollis A. (2009) Albany judge blocks vaccination rule. *New York Times.*
63. Task Force on Community Preventive Services. (2005) Recommendations to improve targeted vaccination coverage among high-risk adults. *Am J Prev Med* **28**: 231–237.
64. Stein R. (2009) Preparing for swine flu's return. *The Washington Post.*

Chapter 5

The Second Wave of the Pandemic (Mid-August 2009 through May 2010)

"Do not dwell in the past, do not dream of the future, concentrate the mind on the present moment."

Buddha

5.1 The Second Wave of the Pandemic

5.1.1 *Epidemiology and Impact of the Second Wave*

A KEY POINT: The history of pandemics suggests that second waves have a substantially greater impact on the world's population than the first wave. This was certainly the case in many countries in the Northern Hemisphere during the 2009 pandemic where the incidence of illness, hospitalizations and deaths increased during the second wave. Surge capacity was strained to the limit in the outpatient and inpatient settings in many medical centers, particularly in the emergency departments and ICU settings. Some of these medical centers had to invoke special measures such as setting up emergency tent facilities in order to provide care to all those seeking medical assistance. However, similar to the first wave, the rate of infection, hospitalization and death during the second wave varied substantially not only between developed and developing countries, but also amongst developed countries and various communities in the same country. In many countries the number of deaths was lower than normally seen with seasonal influenza, but the number of life years lost was high since most of the deaths were occurring in young to middle-aged adults instead of the elderly.

5.1.1.1 *Worldwide*

By September 2009, seven months after the 2009 H1N1 virus had first been detected in Mexico, the world had experienced the first wave of the pandemic during the spring and summer in the Northern Hemisphere and the fall and winter in the Southern Hemisphere. During this time the 2009 H1N1 virus had spread to most, if not all, countries in the world. The intensity of the disease had varied quite widely, with the experiences being relatively mild in some countries and more severe in others.

By October 2009, the second wave of the pandemic was underway in multiple countries in the Northern Hemisphere. By this time there had been >400,000 confirmed cases and almost 5,000 deaths reported. The actual number of cases was believed to be much higher since most countries had stopped trying to identify or confirm suspected cases.

Many of the countries in temperate regions of the Southern Hemisphere had now passed the peak of the first wave, but disease continued to be reported in various countries throughout the Southern Hemisphere. Interestingly, East Asia was one of the few parts of the world where an H3N2 seasonal influenza virus was still causing disease, but even in this part of the world, the 2009 H1N1 virus was the dominant influenza strain. Tropical regions throughout Asia and South America continued to experience geographically regional or widespread influenza activity and were reporting increasing or sustained high levels of respiratory disease. In contrast, many of the tropical regions of Central America and the Caribbean were reporting a declining trend in the level of respiratory diseases.

An increased risk of severe disease due to the 2009 H1N1 virus was occurring in minority populations. In Australia, New Zealand and Canada, the indigenous populations infected with the 2009 H1N1 virus had a 3–8 times increased risk of hospitalization and death.[65] In the USA, American Indians and Alaskan Natives infected with the 2009 H1N1 virus had a mortality rate four times higher than persons in all other racial/ethnic populations. The exact reasons for the increased incidence of severe morbidity and mortality remain to be determined. However, it is likely that the high incidence of chronic diseases, including asthma and diabetes, as well as healthcare disparities due to the poor socioeconomic conditions of these populations, contributed substantially to this increased risk.[66]

The surge capacity in various communities within many countries proved to be inadequate during the second wave due to a substantial increase in patients requiring outpatient and inpatient care, especially those needing to be admitted to an ICU. The increased number of patients with pandemic influenza also impacted the ability to provide care for those with other illnesses. Triage plans were formulated in many medical centers to help decide which patients would be seen on a given day and, for those requiring inpatient care, which unit they would be admitted to (e.g., ICU). When situations arose due to scarce medical resources (e.g., ICU beds, ventilators, etc.), some medical centers gave preference to those whose medical condition suggested that they would obtain greatest benefit from these resources, while in other centers it was on a first-come, first-served basis. These decisions about triage were most problematic in developing countries, but were also present in developed countries including the USA where most states had inadequate surge capacity (see Section 5.1.1.2 for details). Overall the hospitalization rate declined with age, while the death rate was highest in those >25 years of age (Fig. 21).

By the end of 2009, the second wave had run its course in a number of countries in the Northern Hemisphere, but had not yet started in the Southern Hemisphere (Fig. 22). Worldwide, approximately ~75% of influenza cases were due to the 2009 H1N1 virus and most of the other cases were due to influenza B. In temperate and tropical regions of the Southern Hemisphere, there were sporadic cases of 2009 H1N1 still occurring, but the second wave had not yet begun. In North America the second wave of influenza was on the decline. Transmission of disease was widespread in parts of Western, Central and Southeastern Europe as well as in East and West Asia, but the overall rates were low or declining. The limited data from North Africa suggested that 2009 H1N1 virus transmission was widespread, but that it had recently peaked in most areas. In the first quarter of 2010, most countries in the Northern and Southern Hemispheres had been through one or two waves and influenza activity was decreasing in most areas of the globe, except for the southern part of Asia and West

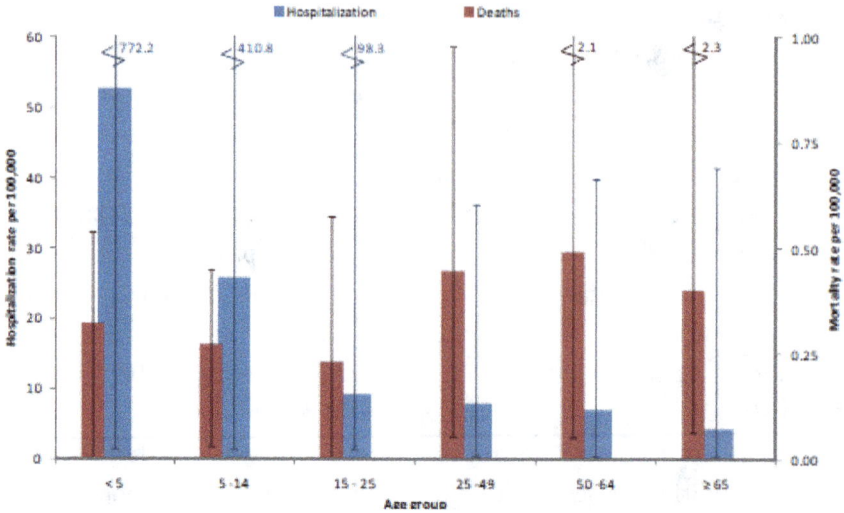

Fig. 21. Population-based rates of hospitalization and death. This figure was taken from a slide presentation, "Update on the Epidemiology of Influenza Viruses", by Dr. Anthony Mounts at the SAGE meeting on April 14, 2010 (http://www.who.int/immunization/sage/previous_april2010/en/index1.html).

Africa where disease activity was just beginning. In the 12 months since the first patients with 2009 H1N1 infection had been detected in Mexico, 213 countries had reported laboratory-confirmed cases of disease due to this virus.[68]

Many experts were concerned that as more people developed immunity against the 2009 H1N1 virus, the virus could mutate in a manner that would enhance its survival and ability to cause more severe disease. In November 2009, the WHO reported that a D222G mutation in the 2009 H1N1 virus had been detected in patients from seven countries in the Northern and Southern Hemispheres. The mutation was predicted to cause increased binding to lower airway cells and this raised the concern that this might result in increased virulence of the virus. The mutation appeared to be a naturally occurring, low-frequency event, and there was no evidence of person-to-person transmission. The virus remained fully sensitive to oseltamivir and zanamivir and the pandemic vaccine afforded protection against this mutated virus. Overall, the genetic makeup of the 2009 H1N1

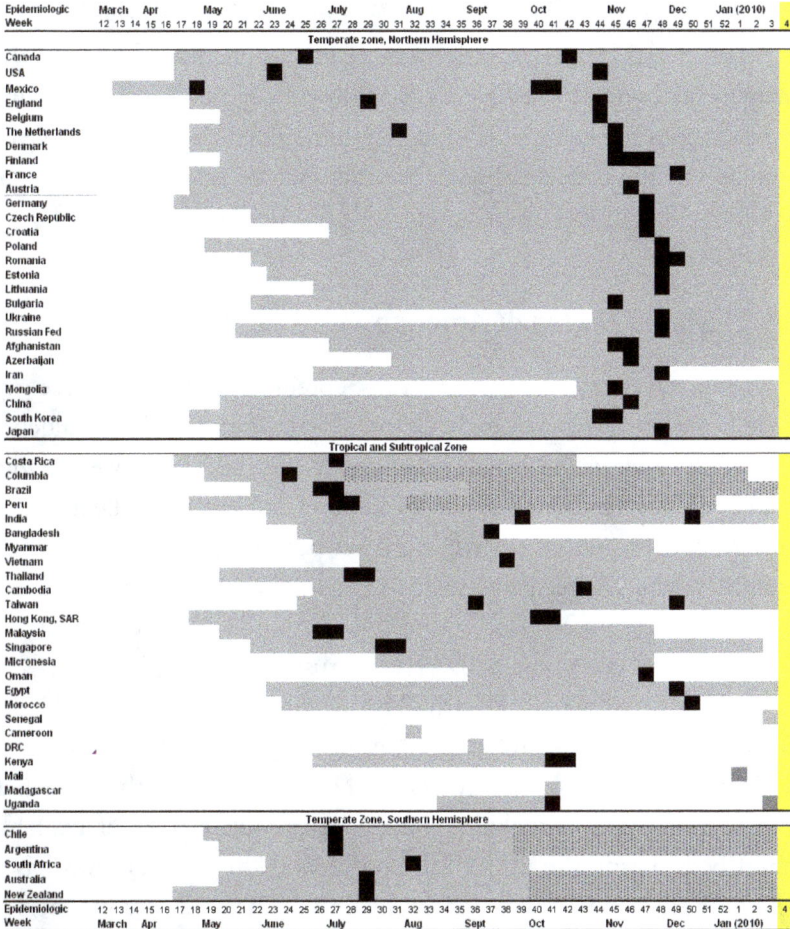

Fig. 22. The time course of the 2009 pandemic in those countries where surveillance systems were in place to detect the virus in patients. The top, middle and bottom parts of the figure depict countries in the northern temperate, tropic and subtropic, and southern temperate zones, respectively. Data from the tropical regions are less robust due to inadequate surveillance capacity in many of these countries. This figure was taken from a slide presentation, "Update on the Epidemiology of Influenza Viruses", by Dr. Anthony Mounts at the SAGE meeting on April 14, 2010 (http://www.who.int/immunization/sage/previous_april2010/en/index1.html).

virus underwent minimal change during the first and second waves of the pandemic. Thus, the wide disparities in hospitalization rates and deaths seen between and within countries were unlikely due to an increase in the virulence of the virus. Other factors, including the incidence of underlying chronic diseases and healthcare infrastructure capabilities, no doubt played a role, but the importance of each or other factors as an explanation for this difference in disease severity remains to be determined.

5.1.1.2 *United States of America*

The second wave started in the USA in September 2009 and disease was widespread in most states by early October. Data from the CDC Influenza Surveillance Network indicated that influenza-like illness rates were higher in October than they had been at the peak of the last five influenza seasons. Compared to the first wave, a greater percentage of the population became ill and a greater percentage of those who were hospitalized had no underlying disease. By mid-October, more than 21,000 hospitalizations and 2,400 deaths due to the 2009 H1N1 virus had been reported.

The Trust for America's Health (TFAH) released a new report "H1N1 Challenges Ahead" in October 2009, indicating that 35% of Americans were likely to get sick from the 2009 H1N1 virus by the time the pandemic was over.[69] The report concluded that 15 states could run out of available hospital beds during the peak of the outbreak. This estimate was based on the FluSurge model developed by the CDC. The predicted numbers of people who would become ill ranged from a high of 12.9 million in California to a low of 186,434 in Wyoming. The number of people hospitalized ranged from a high of 168,025 in California to a low of 2,485 in Wyoming. The report noted that many states could face shortages of beds or need to reduce the number of non-influenza–related elective admissions due to limited hospital bed availability.

The 2009 H1N1 virus was still primarily affecting children and young and middle-aged adults during the second wave. Those >65 years of age became ill less frequently. Preliminary data on 500 children confirmed that those <2 years of age were being hospitalized at a rate 250% higher than any other age group. Confirmed deaths due to the 2009 H1N1 virus had now occurred in >80 children with over half of these deaths occurring in those with neuromuscular diseases while ~30% occurred in children with no risk factors.[70,71]

Influenza activity in the USA had declined substantially to near seasonal baselines by December 2009. Influenza-like illness-related medical visits decreased to 2.6% (the national baseline for influenza-like illness-related visits is 2.3%) and only 11 states were still reporting widespread influenza activity. The proportion of deaths attributed to pneumonia and influenza (P&I) continued to decrease, but remained elevated for the time of year. The P&I had been higher than expected for 11 consecutive weeks.

At the ACIP meeting on February 24 the CDC provided the following updated estimates on the impact of the 2009 pandemic in the USA:

- 57 million cases had occurred with 19 million being in children.
- 257,000 hospitalizations had occurred with the rate being highest in the youngest children and declining with age.
- 58% of children and 85% of adults who were hospitalized had underlying conditions. The relative frequency of the various conditions were similar to that noted in wave 1 (Table 9).
- Over 11,000 deaths occurred, with the lowest rate in the youngest children. However, the total number of deaths that were reported in children (262 childhood deaths as of the time of the February ACIP meeting) was substantially greater than in any previous year since these data were first collected during the 2003–2004 influenza season when 152 pediatric deaths were documented.
- Racial and ethnic disparities with severe outcomes continued to be noted, including a higher proportion of deaths in African Americans compared to all other ethnic populations.

At this point in time the estimated number of hospitalizations due to the 2009 H1N1 virus and a typical influenza season were similar (246,000 for the 2009 pandemic versus 226,000 for a typical influenza season), but the

Table 14. USA Excess Mortality and Years of Life Lost Due to the 2009 H1N1 Virus[*]

Event	Number of Deaths[†]	Mean Age of Deaths (yrs)	Years of Life Lost[†]
2009 pandemic	7,500–44,100[¶] 12,000 (8,500–17,600)[††]	37.4	334,000–1,973,000 463,000 (328,000–680,000)
1968 pandemic	86,000[+]	62.2	1,693,000
1957 pandemic	150,600[+]	64.6	2,698,000
1918 pandemic	1,272,300[+]	27.2	63,718,000
Average A/H3N2 season, 1979–2001	47,800[+]	75.7	594,000

[*]This table was created and published by Viboud et al.[71]
[†]The estimates are adjusted to 2000 population.
[¶]Range is an estimate of excess P&I deaths (lower) and all-cause deaths (upper), based on projections from the 122-city mortality surveillance done in the USA.
[††]Estimates based on the CDC's probabilistic estimates, using 2009 pandemic survey data, which is different from the CDC's excess mortality method for measuring seasonal influenza burden.
[+]Estimates based on the excess mortality approach applied to final national vital statistics and adjusted to the 2000 population age structure.

estimated number of deaths was substantially less (11,000 versus 36,000, respectively). However, the absolute number of deaths for young adults exceeded by 50% those that occurred in the 1968 pandemic and by more than threefold that seen for seasonal influenza.[71] An estimate of the number of years of life lost in the 2009 pandemic compared to seasonal influenza and in the 1918, 1957 and 1968 pandemics was recently published by Viboud et al.[72] and shown in Table 14.

5.1.1.3 *Local communities*

Many local communities found that their emergency rooms and intensive care units were overwhelmed. As the second wave moved across the

USA, communities experienced a surge in outpatient visits for a 4–8-week period sometime during the fall. Many medical centers were inundated with inpatients infected with the 2009 H1N1 virus, and in some of these centers, >50% of the adult and pediatric ICU beds were occupied by patients infected with the 2009 H1N1 virus. These patients often required ventilators, and some needed oscillators (high-frequency ventilators) or extracorporeal membrane oxygenation (ECMO — a technology that allows the heart and lung functions of a patient to be done by a machine outside the patient's body) for weeks or longer. Despite the severity of disease in those requiring ECMO, ~80% of the patients survived.[73] Some patients were admitted to the ICU due to secondary bacterial pneumonias, but the majority (49–72%) had acute viral pneumonia along with the acute onset of ARDS, often with renal insufficiency and hepatic dysfunction.[74]

The number of patients with influenza-like illness seen in the Wake Forest University Baptist Medical Center outpatient facilities, including the emergency department, more than doubled from the week of September 22 through November 6, 2010, compared to previous and subsequent weeks. By the end of the second wave, a total of 169 patients with laboratory-proven 2009 H1N1 infection had been admitted to the Medical Center's hospital. Twenty of the 79 pediatric patients (25%) required care in the PICU, including ventilation, and five of these children required ventilatory support and one required ECMO for many weeks. Twenty-four of the 90 adult patients (27%) were cared for in the ICU and 16 of these patients required ventilatory support and two needed ECMO. There were no pediatric deaths, but five adults, all with high-risk conditions, died of primary viral pneumonia or secondary bacterial infections. This surge of patients requiring ICU care resulted in referring physicians having increased difficulty getting their critically ill patients transferred to tertiary medical centers. The patients turned down for transfer included not only those with influenza-related problems, but those with other types of condition.

5.1.2 *Prevention and Treatment of 2009 H1N1 Infections*

A KEY POINT: Vaccination of the population was the cornerstone of the worldwide stategy to mitigate the impact of the 2009 pandemic. In many countries, the second wave was resulting in a greater percentage of the population being infected with the 2009 H1N1 virus. The first doses of the 2009 pandemic vaccine were just beginning to be released and a critical question was whether the vaccine could be produced and administered to enough people in time to decrease the impact of the pandemic. By the time that the second wave was over in the USA, ~47 million people had been infected, >200,000 people had been hospitalized and ~11,000 people had died. Unfortunately, in Northern Hemisphere countries, only a small percentage of the total amount of H1N1 vaccine that would eventually be produced was available by the time the second wave had peaked.

5.1.2.1 *Vaccines*

5.1.2.1.1 Worldwide use of pandemic and seasonal vaccines

At the SAGE October 28, 2009 meeting the current status of pandemic worldwide vaccine production and use was reviewed. Intramuscular and intranasal monovalent pandemic influenza vaccines, using the A/California/7/2009 H1N1 virus, were now starting to become available. Over 20 developed countries had started to offer the limited quantities of available pandemic vaccine to certain prioritized groups. In all of these countries, HCWs and those at highest risk for developing severe disease were prioritized to get the vaccine first, but in many of these countries, the quantity of vaccine available forced them to prioritize who in the high-risk groups would get the vaccine (Table 15).

The anticipated worldwide production capacity for pandemic vaccine had been revised downward from 5 billion to 1.3 billion doses of

H1N1 vaccine in 12 months (slide presentation "Global Pandemic Vaccine Production and Preliminary Analysis of Deployment of H1N1 Pandemic Vaccine Donated by WHO" by Dr. Marie-Paule Kieny at the April 14, 2010 SAGE meeting [http://www.who.int/immunization/sage/previous_april2010/en/index1.html]). Ninety-five low- to middle-income countries

Table 15. Pandemic Vaccine Prioritization Plans of Various Countries as of October 26, 2009*

Country	First Day of Proposed Vaccine Use	Target Group	Manufacturers
Australia	Sep 30, 2009	— pregnant women — parents/guardians of infants <6 mth — people with high-risk conditions — people with severe obesity — indigenous Australians — HCWs — community care workers	CSL
Austria	Oct 26, 2009 Nov 9, 2009	— HCWs — people with high-risk conditions	Baxter
Belgium	Oct 18, 2009	— HCWs	
Brazil	Jan 2010	— HCWs — children	Butantan Institute
Canada	Oct 28, 2009	— people with chronic medical — conditions <65 yr — pregnant women — children 6 mth to 4 yr — people in remote/isolated locales — HCWs — household contacts/caregivers of individuals at high risk and cannot be immunized (e.g., infants <6 mth, immunosuppressed patients)	GlaxoSmithKline (GSK)

(Continued)

Table 15. (Continued)

Country	First Day of Proposed Vaccine Use	Target Group	Manufacturers
China	Sep 21, 2009	— 200,000 participants in National Day parade — students aged 5–19 yr — hospital patients — HCWs — soldiers, police officers — railway, airline and border-control workers	10 domestic companies
China (Tapei)	Nov 1, 2009	— people in areas hit by Typhoon Morakot — medical personnel	Novartis (5 million)
	Nov 2, 2009	— infants 6–12 mth	ADImmune Corp. (10 million)
Finland	Oct 22, 2009	— HCWs — pregnant women	n/a+
France	Oct 20, 2009	— HCWs — people with high-risk conditions <65 yr — pregnant women	GSK Novartis Sanofi Pasteur
	Nov 2009	— babies and small children — people with high-risk conditions ≥65 yr	
Germany	Oct 26, 2009	— high-risk groups — HCWs	n/a
Hungary	Sep 29, 2009	— children — pregnant women — people with high-risk conditions <60 yr — HCWs	Omninvest Kft.
	n/a	— general public	
Israel	n/a	— HCWs — people with high-risk conditions 10–65 yr	Sanofi Pasteur Novartis GSK

(*Continued*)

Table 15. (Continued)

Country	First Day of Proposed Vaccine Use	Target Group	Manufacturers
Japan	Oct 19, 2009	— HCWs — pregnant women — children	GSK Novartis 4 domestic companies
Mexico	Oct 2009	n/a	Vaccine filled/ finished domestically; bulk from Sanofi Pasteur GSK
Portugal	Oct 26, 2009	— HCWs — pregnant women — people with high-risk conditions	n/a
Qatar	Nov 2009 Jan 2010	— students — general public	n/a
Romania	Dec 2009	n/a	Cantacuzino (domestic)
Russia	Dec 2009	— HCWs — people working in vital sectors	n/a
Singapore	End 2009	— HCWs — people with high-risk conditions	GSK
Spain	Nov 15, 2009	— HCWs — people working in vital sectors — people with high-risk conditions	GSK Novartis
Republic of Korea	Oct 26, 2009	n/a	Green Cross (domestic)
Sweden	Oct 12, 2009	— HCWs	n/a
UAE	n/a	— HCWs — pregnant women — all those 6 mth to 24 yr	GSK Novartis

(Continued)

Table 15. (*Continued*)

Country	First Day of Proposed Vaccine Use	Target Group	Manufacturers
UK	Oct 22, 2009	— childcare personnel — people with high-risk conditions 25–64 yr — pregnant women — people in current seasonal influenza vaccine clinical at-risk groups — household contacts of people with compromised immune systems	GSK Baxter
US	Oct 5, 2009	— HCWs — pregnant women — people caring for those <6 mth — all those 6 mth to 24 yr — people with high-risk conditions 25–64 yr	MedImmune Sanofi Pasteur CSL Novartis

*Adapted from a presentation made at the SAGE October 28, 2009 meeting (http://www.who.int/immunization/sage/previous_October2009/en/index1.html).
n/a – information not available.

that would otherwise not have access to pandemic vaccines were eligible based on need to receive support through the WHO pandemic vaccine initiative. To minimize disruption of healthcare services, the WHO would provide each developing country with enough doses of the pandemic vaccine to immunize at least its HCWs (2% of its population), as recommended by SAGE on July 7, 2009. The delivery of the vaccine to eligible countries was expected to occur over the period of November 2009–February 2010.

The WHO had ~180 million doses of the monovalent pandemic vaccine in its stockpile by December 2009. Manufacturing, political and logistical problems had caused delays and prevented earlier shipments of the vaccine. The WHO now began distributing the vaccine to about three dozen developing countries, with Azerbaijan and Mongolia receiving the first shipments. Since the first wave of the pandemic was over in the Southern Hemisphere, the WHO sent the vaccine to countries in the Northern Hemisphere that were still being impacted by the second wave of the pandemic. The WHO distributed vaccines only to those developing nations that requested a shipment, agreed to the WHO's terms and conditions of use, and implemented a national plan to ensure HCWs, followed by pregnant women and other populations, as recommended by SAGE, were immunized if enough vaccine was available. The process of distributing the vaccine to developing countries moved forward slowly due to problems with vaccine availability and logistical issues in various countries. By the end of February 2010, the WHO had delivered 2,205,600 vaccine doses to 7 countries and by the end of March, 15,206,800 vaccine doses had been delivered to 29 countries (data presented at the SAGE April 2010 meeting).

A further goal was to provide each of these 95 countries with enough vaccine to immunize up to 10% of its population that was at highest risk for serious morbidity and mortality due to the 2009 H1N1 virus. To achieve this goal would require more than 200 million doses of the pandemic vaccine to be available over the next 6–12 months, and the WHO continued to work with developed countries and the vaccine industry to free up as much vaccine as possible for use in developing countries. By the time of the April 2010 SAGE meeting, 13 donor countries, the Gates Foundation and five donor manufacturers had pledged 190 million doses of the monovalent pandemic vaccine, 74.5 million syringes and $46 million for operation support to help with logistical issues. Thirty-one countries had received the vaccine and an additional 20 countries had been approved to get vaccine shipments based on their readiness to start vaccinating their population.

Pandemic vaccines (live attenuated, adjuvanted and non-adjuvanted inactivated vaccine products) produced in various countries had been licensed in their respective countries for use as a single-dose schedule for those ≥10 years of age (the only exception was with the vaccine made by Roche where two doses of the vaccine were still required). For children

6 months to 9 years of age, the SAGE recommended that until more data were available for the different formulations of vaccine, children in this age group should receive two doses of the vaccine. SAGE noted that in the interests of public health, vaccine supplies should be used to give first doses to as many children as possible, with second doses to follow as further supplies became available.

Subsequently, initial results of NIH trials examining the response of children to one of the 2009 H1N1 monovalent unadjuvanted vaccines became available.[75] Results from a study of 583 children showed that only 25% of children between the ages of 6 and 35 months and 55% of children between ages 3 and 9 years were adequately protected by one dose of the vaccine. The protection rate rose to 100% among 6–35-month-olds and 94% for 3–9-year-olds after receiving a second dose of the vaccine. In contrast, a study using a different monovalent unadjuvanted vaccine made in Australia found that 161 of 174 (92.5%) infants and children had an adequate immune response to one dose of the vaccine. Given these conflicting results, the known variability that occurs when different laboratories measure HA titers on the same samples, and the existing data on seasonal influenza vaccines that indicated that children <9 years of age needed two doses of vaccine during the first season that they received the vaccine, most authorities continued to recommend that two doses of the 2009 pandemic vaccine be given to children <10 years of age.[76]

Clinical trials investigating the feasibility of co-administration of seasonal and pandemic vaccines were performed. When seasonal and pandemic vaccines were both inactivated, or when one was inactivated and the other was live attenuated, SAGE recommended that they could be co-administered. SAGE concurred with the CDC recommendation that live attenuated seasonal and live attenuated pandemic vaccines should not be co-administered and should be separated by ≥28 days.

Influenza vaccines had been used in pregnant women for over a decade in many countries due to the increased risk of these women for hospitalization due to seasonal influenza. A study of unadjuvanted pandemic vaccine in 50 pregnant women in their second or third trimesters showed that 92% developed sufficient immunity 21 days after receiving a 15 ug dose of vaccine, leading officials to believe that one dose of vaccine is sufficient. Reproductive toxicity studies conducted in pregnant animal models with non-adjuvanted and adjuvanted pandemic TIV and LAIV had not suggested any harmful effects with respect to the pregnant women or fetus and regulatory agencies allowed the use of the 2009 pandemic vaccine in pregnant women. Based on these facts, and in view of the substantial risk for severe outcomes in pregnant women infected with the 2009 H1N1 virus, SAGE recommended that, in the absence of a specific contraindication by the regulatory authority in a given country, any licensed pandemic vaccine could be used to protect pregnant women.

In late September 2009, just as the pandemic vaccine was about to be used in various countries, a report from Canada suggested that people who got the 2008–2009 seasonal influenza vaccine were more prone to get infected with the 2009 H1N1 virus.[77] The study suggested that people vaccinated against seasonal influenza were twice as likely to become infected with the 2009 H1N1 virus. This finding was quite unexpected and led various countries including the USA, United Kingdom and Australia to review their own data but they were unable to find any evidence that supported these findings.[78]

Despite the inconsistency between the data from Canada and these other countries, five Canadian provinces indicated that they planned to delay part of their 2009–2010 seasonal influenza immunization program until the pandemic vaccine had been offered to their targeted groups. Public health authorities in these provinces indicated that they would offer the seasonal influenza vaccine starting in mid-October to people ≥65 years and to residents of long-term care facilities, but in November, when the pandemic vaccine would be available in Canada, the seasonal program would be stopped and efforts switched over to giving the pandemic vaccine. By the end of 2009, ~45% of the Canadian population had chosen to get the pandemic vaccine. With the second wave on the decline, there was little additional demand for the pandemic vaccine and Canadian authorities reinitiated the seasonal influenza vaccination campaign in early 2010.

Since the onset of the use of the monovalent pandemic vaccine in October 2009, intense safety surveillance was being conducted worldwide by multiple public health (e.g., WHO and CDC) and regulatory entities (e.g., European Medicines Agency and Food and Drug Administration). By the end of March 2010, >350 million doses of pandemic vaccine had been administered worldwide with no unusual safety concerns noted. These data were taken from a slide presentation, "Update on H1N1 Vaccine Immunogenicity, Safety and Effectiveness", by Dr. David Woods at the April 14, 2010 SAGE meeting (http://www.who.int/immunization/ sage/previous_april2010/en/index1.html). There had been two recalls of certain lots of Sanofi's and MedImmune's vaccines, but this was due to tests that showed the potency of these lots had decreased below the pre-specified levels and not due to safety issues.

Despite the encouraging safety data, <10% of the populations of the United Kingdom, Ireland, Italy, Germany and France had received the 2009 pandemic vaccine by December 2009 compared to the ~20% influenza vaccination rate that occurred during a typical epidemic season. The low uptake of the pandemic vaccine was attributed to concerns about safety, mortality rates that were lower than originally predicted, and an already declining incidence of illness during the second wave in these countries. By this time the overall mortality rate was estimated to be <0.5%, but there was a wide range of estimates that reflected the uncertainty regarding case ascertainment and the actual number of people infected.[73] The United Kingdom had 10 million doses of vaccine available, but only 1.6 million of 9.3 million high-risk individuals had been vaccinated. Overall, this amounted to <2% of the nation's population of 60 million. In Italy and France, the percentage of their population who had gotten the vaccine by this time was even lower. Some of the countries cancelled up to 50% of the vaccine doses they had previously ordered (National Network for Immunization Information Newsbriefs, December 10, 2009, http://www.immunizationinfo.org/).

5.1.2.1.2 United States of America

The FDA had approved for use in the USA, the unadjuvanted intramuscular monovalent pandemic vaccine and the intranasal unadjuvanted live adapted monovalent vaccine. These vaccines were made by the same companies (CSL, Novartis, Sanofi Pasteur, GlaxoSmithKline and Med-Immune) that already supplied the USA with seasonal TIV and LAIV vaccines and were manufactured using the same formulations and processes.

To assess the safety profile of the pandemic vaccine, the CDC reviewed vaccine safety from 3,783 reports received through the USA Vaccine Adverse Event Reporting System (VAERS) through November 2009 and electronic data from 438,376 persons vaccinated in managed-care organizations that are part of the Vaccine Safety Datalink (VSD), a large, population-based database with administrative and diagnostic data. No substantial differences between the 2009 H1N1 and seasonal influenza vaccines were noted in the proportion or types of serious adverse events reported. No increase in any adverse events undergoing surveillance was detected in the VSD database. Ten cases of GBS had been reported and this was fewer than the number of cases that would be expected to occur in the general population who had not yet been vaccinated. The CDC and other USA government agencies also used multiple other systems to monitor H1N1 vaccine safety (Table 16).

In late April 2010, USA health officials reported that for the first time, data that five of the above noted detection networks the government was using to monitor vaccine safety suggested there might be a very small increase risk from the pandemic vaccine of GBS, Bell's palsy (a temporary facial paralysis) and thrombocytopenia (low platelets). The officials stressed that it was too early to tell whether the vaccine was causing a small increased risk of the above noted conditions or whether there was some other explanation (e.g., physicians identifying more cases because of the intensive effort to pinpoint any safety problems with the vaccine). Given how closely the vaccine's safety was being monitored, it had been anticipated that some possible adverse events would be detected, but turn out to be false alarms.

Based on the preliminary report about these potential side effects, the USA Health and Human Services Department's National Vaccine Advisory Committee, which had been charged with monitoring the vaccine's

Table 16. Surveillance Systems Used to Monitor the Safety of the 2009 H1N1 Pandemic Vaccine in the USA*

System	Federal Agency	Description	Approximate USA Population Monitored
Vaccine Adverse Event Reporting System (VAERS)	CDC, Food and Drug Administration	HCWs and manufacturers are required to report to VAERS certain adverse events in vaccinees. HCWs and the public can report other adverse events voluntarily. VAERS enables early detection of new, rare or unusual patterns of adverse events that can be investigated using other methods. Enhancements to VAERS include providing information on influenza vaccination record cards, advertising in medical journals, using state vaccine safety coordinators, and increased report processing capacity.	Entire population
Vaccine Safety Datalink (VSD)	CDC	Uses administrative data and electronic medical records to collect information on vaccinations and healthcare encounters to monitor vaccine safety. VSD monitors H1N1 vaccine safety using historical and other appropriate comparison groups. Data is analyzed weekly.	9.5 million
Population-based active surveillance for Guillain–Barré syndrome (GBS)	CDC	CDC and Emerging Infections Program sites actively identify GBS cases, using a network of neurologists and collaboration with the American Academy of Neurology.	45 million

(Continued)

Table 16. (Continued)

System	Federal Agency	Description	Approximate USA Population Monitored
Real-Time Immunization Monitoring System	CDC	Allows vaccinees to register online at the time of vaccination; solicits reports of post-vaccination adverse events with e-mails on the day of vaccination and 7 days and 42 days after vaccination.	Entire population
Post-Licensure Rapid Immunization Safety Monitoring	National Vaccine Program Office, CDC, Food and Drug Administration	Active surveillance using electronic billing, diagnostic and vaccination data from state vaccine registries and large health plans in several states.	30 million (17 million with registry-enhanced data)
Defense Medical Surveillance System	USA Department of Defense	An executive information, electronic medical record system containing longitudinal data on USA active duty military personnel.	1.4 million
Veterans Affairs Adverse Drug Event Reporting System (VA ADERS)	USA Department of Veterans Affairs	VA health system, including veterans and employees.	1.2 million
Medicare data systems	Centers for Medicare and Medicaid Services	National Claims History File and Enrollment Database for persons enrolled in fee-for-service Medicare; used for retrospective and prospective vaccine safety studies, primarily among persons aged ≥ 65 years.	38 million

(*Continued*)

Table 16. (*Continued*)

System	Federal Agency	Description	Approximate USA Population Monitored
Indian Health Service electronic health records	Indian Health Service	Can conduct enhanced VAERS surveillance and provide signal detection.	1.4 million
Vaccines and Medications in Pregnancy Surveillance System	Biomedical Advanced Research and Development Authority	A collaboration of academic and professional investigators that can monitor the relationship between receipt of H1N1 2009 monovalent vaccines, seasonal influenza vaccines and antiviral medications in pregnancy and subsequent maternal and fetal outcomes.	Prospective cohort study (1,100). Case-control surveillance (2,000)
Clinical Immunization Safety Assessment Network	CDC	Collaboration between CDC and six academic sites with vaccine safety expertise provides broad consultation on clinical issues that arise during safety monitoring, including review of possible GBS and anaphylaxis reports.	Entire population

*Adapted from Table 3 of "Influenza A (H1N1 2009 Monovalent Vaccines — United States, October 1–November 24, 2009", MMWR (2009) **58**(early release): 1–6.

safety, decided to follow up on these findings. The Committee noted that the data suggesting a problem was not strong and that further analysis might well show no increased risk of these side effects. Additionally, they pointed out that even if one or more of these side effects were caused by the vaccine, they were occurring on a very infrequent basis (e.g., the Committee reported the vaccine at most could be causing one extra case of GBS per one million people vaccinated). Thus, even if the adverse events turned out to be real, the danger from the 2009 H1N1 virus itself remained far greater than that from the vaccine.

For the 2009–2010 seasonal influenza vaccine, there was greater demand than anticipated and mismatches between the supply and demand occurred in many communities. By the end of October 2009, the CDC estimated that 85 million Americans already had received the seasonal influenza vaccine, up from 61 million at the same time in 2008. The reason why the uptake of the seasonal vaccine was greater than in previous years was, at least in part, due to the extensive media coverage about the pandemic and the recommendations that everyone be vaccinated with both the seasonal and pandemic vaccines. Additionally, there was also a shortage of seasonal influenza vaccines in some communities and media coverage of this likely led to increased demand for the vaccine. Four of the five seasonal influenza vaccine manufacturers licensed in the USA had plants overseas and some were under pressure from the home government not to send the vaccine outside the country. Although manufacturers had produced a total of 114 million doses of the seasonal influenza vaccine for the USA, 24 million doses had yet to be delivered. Various healthcare providers ran out of the vaccine and this situation was not remedied until the later part of November.

The first doses of the monovalent pandemic vaccine were distributed in the first half of October 2009. The actual amount of vaccine being produced was much less than had been predicted due mainly to problems with the poor growth of the 2009 H1N1 virus in eggs and inadequate capacity to rapidly get large quantities of vaccine product to the market. Furthermore, the ability to vaccinate large populations using the public health system was impaired due to substantial cuts in the public health infrastructure that had resulted in ~15,000 jobs being eliminated during the past several years. Due to the economic recession that began in 2008, many states and communities had cut the budgets of their public health departments and this resulted in shortages of personnel who could administer vaccines. This led the CDC to reconsider their plans to deliver the pandemic vaccine through a process that utilized only the public health sector. The CDC continued to have central control over how the pandemic vaccine was distributed, but contracted with McKesson, a private distributor, to transport the vaccine and utilized a combination of the public and private sector to administer the vaccine to the public. Given the small number of vaccine doses available at the time the second wave occurred in the USA, the impact of the public health budget cuts were not a major limiting factor to immunizing the population. Furthermore, since most children and adults in the USA receive their routinely recommended vaccines through the private sector, a public-private model similar to that used during the 2009 pandemic may well be the best way to immunize the public during future pandemics.

In October 2009, as vaccines first became available, most of the doses went to the highest priority group (Fig. 23). However, a survey done of more than 16,000 children and adults found that the overall vaccination rate in the high-priority group was only 30.4% with vaccination rates in the priority subgroups (pregnant women, HCWs, healthy individuals 6 months to 24 years of age, those with underlying risk factors 25–64 years of age and people who have contact with infants) ranging between 24% for people with infant contact and 39% for HCWs. By the end of 2009, 82–91 million doses of the monovalent pandemic vaccine were available in the USA and 72–81 million people had received the vaccine (Fig. 24). Overall, ~29% of the entire USA population >6 months of age had been vaccinated. The vaccine supply was clearly increasing and all states were able to expand their vaccine recommendations to include anyone in the general public who wanted it.

Coverage was higher in children than adults and in a few states as many as 60% of children <10 years of age had received two doses of the vaccine.[79] The better coverage rate amongst children was due in part to the emphasis by many states on getting this population immunized. Coverage did not significantly differ between racial and ethnic groups for children, but in adults coverage was higher in Caucasians compared to the African American and Hispanic populations. More children received both the seasonal and pandemic influenza vaccines than did adults (Fig. 25).

Another problem that occurred was due to a substantial mismatch between the supply versus the demand for the vaccine. This mismatch varied over time in different locales. One of the main factors that contributed to the mismatched supply and demand was the increasing or decreasing

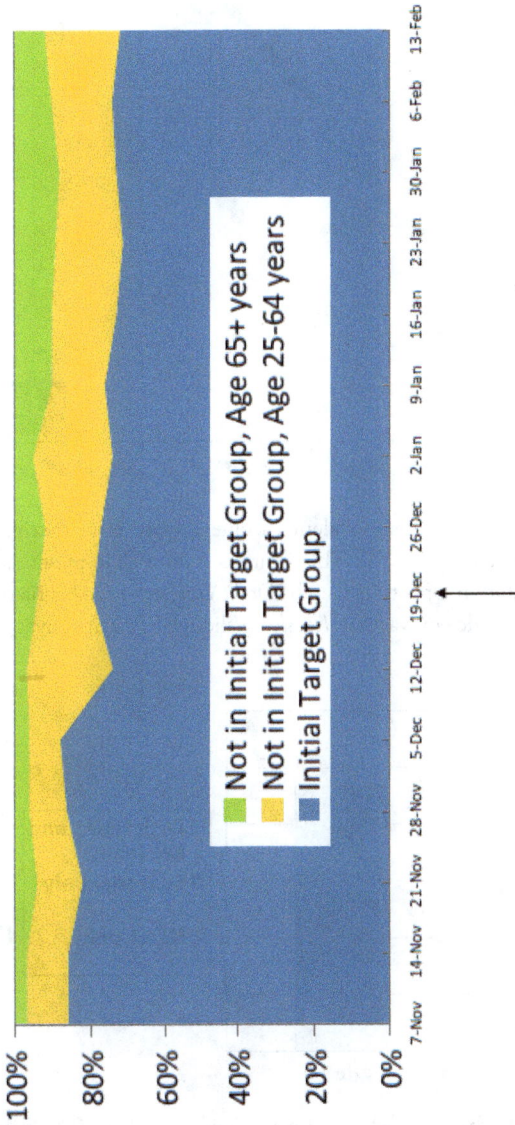

Fig. 23. The percentage of cumulative doses of the 2009 H1N1 monovalent vaccine received by the initial target group (pregnant women, HCWs, those 6 months to 24 years of age, infant contacts and high-risk adults 25–64 years of age). This figure is from a slide presentation, "H1N1 Vaccination Coverage", given by Dr. J. Singleton at the February 24, 2010 ACIP meeting (http://www.cdc.gov/vaccines/recs/acip/slides-feb10.htm#fluvac).

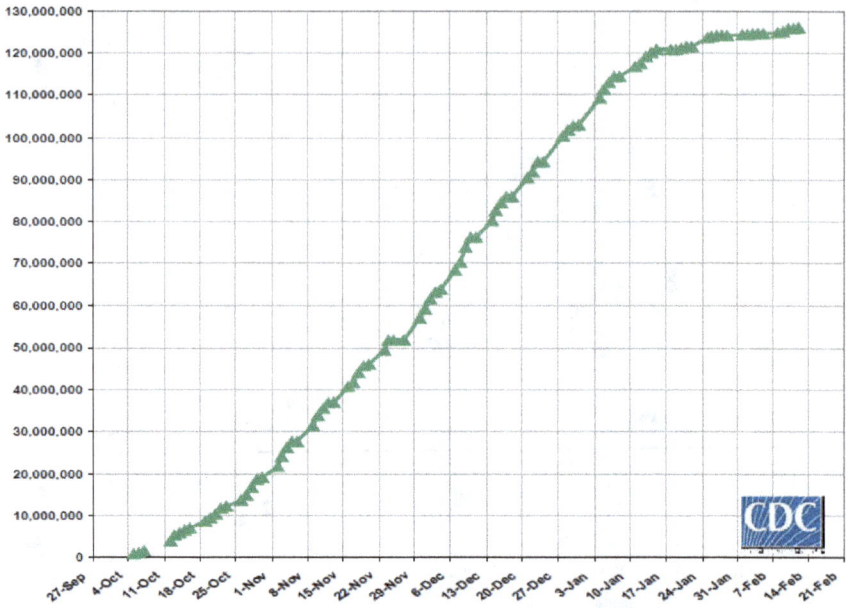

Fig. 24. The number of doses of H1N1 monovalent vaccine shipped from distribution depots to US providers by February 12, 2010. This figure is from a slide presentation, "H1N1 Vaccination Implementation Update", given by Dr. P. Wortley at the February 24, 2010 ACIP meeting (http://www.cdc.gov/vaccines/recs/acip/slides-feb10.htm#fluvac).

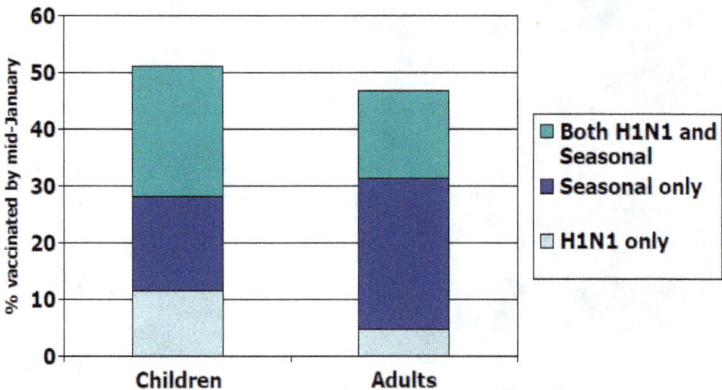

Fig. 25. The percentage of children and adults who received the 2008–2009 seasonal influenza vaccine, the 2009 H1N1 pandemic vaccine or both. This figure is taken from a slide presentation, "H1N1 Vaccination Coverage", by Dr. J. Singleton at the February 24, 2010 ACIP meeting (http://www.cdc.gov/vaccines/recs/acip/slides-feb10.htm#fluvac).

intensity of the second wave at the time the vaccine was being offered in a particular locale and the tone of the messages being delivered by the media (e.g., news articles indicating that the 2009 H1N1 virus was causing only very mild disease versus news articles highlighting deaths due to the virus). In our region, many public health departments had inadequate quantities of vaccine to immunize all those who came to the clinic during the time that the second wave was on the upswing. In contrast, in New York City, only ~5% of the available vaccine was administered in seven clinics that were offering free pandemic vaccine to children and pregnant women despite the fact that a prior telephone survey had indicated that 50% of parents were interested in having their family get the pandemic vaccine.[80]

A survey done by the Harvard School of Public Health in mid-September 2009 found that 52% of people were concerned that someone in their family would get sick from the 2009 H1N1 virus and 70% said they would probably (51% absolutely certain) get the pandemic vaccine when it became available. The major reason for not wanting to get the pandemic vaccine or give their children the pandemic vaccine was a concern about the side effects of the vaccine. Other reasons given in this survey are noted in Table 17.

During this same period, rumors were circulating about illegal or inequitable activities involving the sale of the pandemic vaccine and also preferential delivery of the vaccine to people who were not in the first priority group. A truck delivering the vaccine to Milwaukee, Wisconsin, was hijacked.[81] Reports of the pandemic vaccine being given to individuals who were not in the first priority group included National Hockey League players in Canada being given the vaccine during the period when it was in short supply while high-risk individuals such as pregnant women were having trouble getting the vaccine. Another report suggested that people working in the financial district of New York City were given the vaccine rather than those at greatest risk. This latter story circulated widely, and during the first week of November, Dr. Thomas R. Frieden, Director of the CDC, issued the following letter to officers of state and local health departments emphasizing the need to make certain that the distribution of the pandemic vaccine was given only to those in the first priority group.

Table 17. The Major Reasons Why Adults Said They Were Considering Not Getting the 2009 Pandemic Vaccine for Themselves and/or Their Children*

Reasons Given for Not Getting the Vaccine	Vaccine for Adults (%)	Vaccine for Children (%)
Concern about side effects	30	38
Don't think they are at risk for serious disease	28	27
Medication is available to treat the 2009 H1N1 virus	26	Not noted
Concern about getting 2009 H1N1 infection from the vaccine	21	24
Vaccine is too expensive	20	13
Concern about getting another serious illness from vaccine	20	33
Don't trust public health officials to provide correct information about the vaccine	19	31
Don't think vaccine will be effective	17	23
Don't like shots	16	15
Plan on getting seasonal vaccine and believe this will also protect against the 2009 H1N1 virus	14	12
Healthcare provider said not to get the vaccine	10	7
Too hard to get to location to get the vaccine	8	4

*This table was adapted from a slide presentation "H1N1 Vaccine: Implementation Update", by Dr. Pascale Wortley at the October 22, 2009 ACIP meeting (http://www.cdc.gov/vaccines/recs/ACIP/slides-oct09.htm#fluvac). Data obtained from a survey done by the Harvard Opinion Research Program at the Harvard School of Public Health, September 14–20, 2009.

Dear State/Local Health Officer:

Today we have 35.6 million doses of pandemic vaccine allocated for ordering, with more coming every day. As you know all too well, at present, demand for the vaccine in your communities still exceeds the supply we have received from manufacturers. That means it is more important than ever to focus on ensuring equitable access to the vaccine for the priority groups identified by the Advisory Committee on Immunization Practices: pregnant women, caretakers of infants less than 6 months of age, health care workers, children and adults with health conditions such as asthma or diabetes, and people under the age of 25. These are the people who are most vulnerable to 2009 H1N1 influenza, and it's our job to do everything we can to keep them safe this influenza season.

I know you have been working hard to distribute vaccine to the people who need it most. You are on the front lines of the fight, and no one knows better than you how to reach people in your communities. I especially appreciate the many innovative ways you've found to reach them, including school-located vaccine clinics, special clinics for pregnant women, outreach to children with special needs, and making vaccine available to community- and faith-based organizations serving these high-risk populations. The goal of the H1N1 vaccination program is to protect our population — focusing first on these high-risk groups and ensuring equitable access to the vaccine. While vaccine supplies are still limited, any vaccine distribution decisions that appear to direct vaccine to people outside the identified priority groups have the potential to undermine the credibility of the program. It is important to make it clear to the public that we are all committed to the science-based vaccination recommendations established by the Advisory Committee on Immunization Practices. This may include making clear to the public as well as healthcare providers how the vaccine available to you is being targeted, and the basis for targeting. CDC expects all grantees to ensure that all vaccinators chosen by state and local health departments adhere to those recommendations. Toward that end, and in light of changing projections of vaccine availability, I ask each of you to review your plans immediately and work to ensure that the maximum number of doses is delivered to those at greatest risk as rapidly as possible.

By early December 2009 the second wave of the pandemic was winding down throughout the USA while the quantity of the pandemic vaccine available was substantially increasing. The mismatch between relatively high demand and low supply that had occurred in September and October 2009 was now going in the opposite direction. There were now >85 million doses of the pandemic vaccine available in the USA, but the demand was decreasing. A number of states now had an excess of the vaccine and decided to make it available to everyone including those in priority groups 2 and 3 (Fig. 19). As part of the announcement that the vaccine would now be available to everyone in North Carolina, the State Director of

Public Health emphasized that the pandemic was ongoing and that while the numbers of cases were currently down from the peak of the second wave, the rate of influenza illness was still higher than usual. Furthermore, he predicted that there would likely be a third wave of 2009 H1N1 virus infection. Kathleen Sebelius, the USA Secretary of Health and Human Services, was also encouraging everyone to get the pandemic vaccine, noting that it would lessen the impact, and perhaps even prevent a third wave.

By the end of 2009, the CDC estimated that only 61 million persons (20%) of the USA population had been vaccinated.[82] Despite the initial focus on vaccinating HCWs and those at highest risk of developing severe disease, only 22% and 28%, respectively, of these two groups had received the vaccine. Within the high-risk group, the highest vaccination rate (38%) was in pregnant women and the lowest (12%) in adults 25–64 years of age with high-risk conditions. Tables 18 and 19 show a further breakdown of the vaccination rates in various groups.

By the end of February 2010, as many as 91 million people in the USA had received the 2009 H1N1 vaccine. Given that the second wave was over in the USA at this point there was very little additional demand for the vaccine despite the CDC's continuing recommendation that everyone be vaccinated due to the possibility of a third wave. The pandemic vaccine stockpile now had ~138 million doses of this vaccine and the USA government decided to donate 25 million doses to developing countries. Even with this donation as many as 78 million doses might be discarded due to the expiration date on the various vaccine lots.[83]

5.1.2.2 *Composition of the virus components that should be included in the 2010 influenza seasonal vaccine for the Southern Hemisphere*

At the SAGE October 2009 meeting, consideration was given to which virus strains should be included in the 2010 Southern Hemisphere trivalent seasonal influenza vaccine. During the 2009 influenza season, H3N2 viruses had caused outbreaks in various Southern Hemisphere countries, including China and South Africa, prior to the onset of the pandemic

Table 18. Estimated 2009 H1N1 Monovalent Vaccination Coverage Among USA Residents Aged >6 months, by Age and Priority Group Status — National 2009 H1N1 Flu Survey*

Age Group and Priority Group	USA Population (millions)	Number Surveyed[†]	% Vaccinated (95% CI[§])	Estimated Number of Persons Vaccinated (millions) (95% CI)[¶]
Total ≥6 mths	299	3,023	20.3 (17.2–23.4)	61 (51–70)
6 mths–4 yrs	19	500	33.0 (21.6–44.4)[¶]	6 (4–8)
6 mths–18 yrs	76	1,638	29.4 (23.8–35.0)	22 (18–27)
6 mths–24 yrs	101	1,716	25.9 (20.6–31.2)	26 (21–32)
6 mths–64 yrs	261	2,672	21.7 (18.3–25.1)	57 (48–66)
5–18 yrs	57	1,138	28.1 (21.7–34.5)	16 (12–20)
≥19 yrs	223	1,385	17.3 (13.8–20.8)	39 (31–46)
19–64 yrs	185	1,034	18.6 (14.5–22.7)	34 (27–42)
≥65 years	38	351	11.2 (6.5–15.9)	4 (2–6)
Priority group				
Initial target groups**	160	2,101	27.9 (23.5–32.3)	45 (38–52)
Limited vaccine subset[††]	62	807	37.5 (30.1–44.9)	23 (19–28)

*"Interim results: Influenza A (H1N1) 2009 monovalent vaccination coverage — United States, October 1–December, 2009", MMWR (2010) **59**(02): 44–48. Coverage estimates are based on vaccinations reported as received from October 1, 2009, to the date interviewed.

[†]Excludes 1.5% of respondents with missing vaccination information.

[§]CI — Confidence interval.

[¶]Estimate might be unreliable because of wide CI.

**Pregnant women, persons who live with or provide care for infants aged <6 months, HCWs, emergency medical services personnel, those aged 6 months to 24 years, and persons aged 25–64 years with medical conditions that put them at higher risk for influenza-related complications.

[††]Pregnant women, persons who live with or provide care for infants aged <6 months, HCWs and emergency medical services personnel who have direct contact with patients or infectious material, children aged 6 months to 4 years, and children aged 5–18 years who have medical conditions that put them at higher risk for influenza-related complications.

Table 19. Estimated Influenza A (H1N1) 2009 Monovalent Vaccination Coverage Among USA Residents, by Initial Target Group — Behavioral Risk Factor Surveillance System (BRFSS)[†] and National 2009 H1N1 Flu Survey (NHFS), December 1–27, 2009*

Initial Target Group	Number Surveyed[§]	% Vaccinated (95% CI[¶])
Adults aged 25–64 years with high-risk conditions**	4,044	11.6 (9.9–13.3)
Healthcare personnel[††]	3,329	22.3 (19.6–25.0)
Pregnant women	150	38.0 (24.3–51.7)[§§]
Adults living or caring for infant aged <6 months (NHFS[¶¶])	402	13.9 (9.2–18.6)

*"Interim results: Influenza A (H1N1) 2009 monovalent vaccination coverage — United States, October 1–December, 2009", *MMWR* (2010) **59**(02): 44–48. Coverage estimates are based on vaccinations reported as received from October 1 to the date of the interview.
[†] Includes data from the District of Columbia and all states except Vermont for all adults; excludes Delaware for healthcare personnel and Alaska, Arizona, Delaware and Ohio for pregnant women.
[§] Excludes 2.85% of respondents with missing vaccination information.
[¶] CI — Confidence interval.
**High-risk conditions identified by BRFSS include asthma, diabetes, heart disease and other conditions (lung problems other than asthma, kidney problems, anemia, including sickle cell, or a weakened immune system caused by a chronic illness or by medicines taken for a chronic illness).
[††] Includes persons working in a healthcare setting or providing direct patient care but not in a healthcare setting.
[§§] Estimate might be unreliable because of wide CI.
[¶¶] Data from NHFS interviews conducted during November 29–December 26, 2009. BRFSS did not collect information on this target group.

in this part of the world. Many of these H3N2 viruses were antigenically and genetically similar to A/Brisbane/10/07, the H3N2 strain that had been included in the previous seasonal vaccine. However, an antigenically and genetically distinct H3N2 variant represented by the A/Perth/16/09 virus had emerged and an increasing proportion of H3N2 viruses occurring globally were A/Perth/16/09-like. Therefore, it was recommended that vaccines for use in the 2010 Southern Hemisphere winter influenza seasonal vaccination contain the following strains: A/California/7/2009 (H1N1)-like virus (this is a 2009 H1N1 virus and was the strain used to make the monovalent pandemic vaccine used in the Southern and Northern Hemispheres in 2009), an A/Perth/16/2009 (H3N2)-like virus and a B/Brisbane/60/2008-like virus. The composition of which virus strains to include in the 2010–2011 Northern Hemisphere seasonal influenza vaccine was made in February 2010 and did not differ from the recommendation made for the Southern Hemisphere.[84] Additionally, at the February 24, 2009 ACIP meeting, the universal use of the seasonal influenza vaccine had been updated to include everyone >6 months of age. This new recommendation appeared to be a major expansion of the previous age-based recommendation to vaccinate everyone between 6 months and 18 years, those ≥65 years and all high-risk groups and their contacts. However, in reality this was not the case, since ~85% of the USA population was already recommended to receive the seasonal influenza vaccine based on the previous recommendation.

SAGE also considered whether a bivalent vaccine (strains of A [H3N2] and B) and a separate monovalent pandemic influenza A (H1N1) 2009 vaccine should be produced. SAGE noted the increased programmatic complexities associated with the use of two separate products (bivalent and monovalent influenza vaccines) compared to only using a trivalent vaccine. However, SAGE recognized that the bivalent plus monovalent option was being requested by certain countries in the Southern Hemisphere. This option had the advantage of increasing the availability of pandemic influenza A (H1N1) 2009 vaccine for use in developing countries since it would allow adjuvanted influenza A (H1N1) pandemic vaccine, which required less viral protein per vaccine dose, to be made and used and thereby maximize the availability of the pandemic vaccine. SAGE concluded that both the trivalent and the bivalent plus monovalent options should remain available as an option for the 2010 Southern Hemisphere seasonal influenza vaccination program, subject to national needs. SAGE encouraged Southern Hemisphere countries that choose to use trivalent vaccine to donate any surplus monovalent A pandemic vaccine leftover from the 2009 season to the WHO initiative.

The Australian company CSL, the only manufacturer of influenza vaccines in the Southern Hemisphere, indicated in late November 2009 that production of the 2010 trivalent seasonal influenza vaccine, which included the pandemic strain, would probably be delayed by about one month and was unlikely to be available in Australia until April. The Australian government had ordered 21 million doses of this vaccine from CSL which would provide seasonal flu vaccine for about two-thirds of the Australian market. The delay of availability of the vaccine until April would normally not pose a large problem in the Southern Hemisphere where the influenza season does not usually begin until June or July. However, there was concern that the second wave of the pandemic could occur earlier, since the first wave in the Southern Hemisphere had started in May 2009. An additional problem developed towards the end of April 2010 when Australia's Chief Medical Officer advised providers to stop administering the 2010 seasonal influenza vaccine to children ≤ 5 years of age pending an investigation of reports of fever, convulsions and one death following immunization with several different batches of CSL's vaccine. The trivalent seasonal flu vaccine contained the pandemic H1N1 strain as one of the three viral components, but the advisory did not apply to use of the monovalent H1N1 swine flu vaccine. The investigation was still ongoing at the end of May 2010 (personal communication with Professor David Durrheim, Newcastle University, Australia). A number of other countries, including the USA, decided to make similar recommendations regarding the 2010 trivalent seasonal influenza vaccine.

5.1.2.3 *Antivirals*

During the first and second waves of the pandemic there were adequate supplies of antiviral drugs in most developed countries, but this was not the case in many of the developing countries. Even in developed countries, a number of issues arose including the lack of adequate supplies of the liquid preparation of oseltamivir for young children and the lack of licensed alternative antiviral agents for patients who were infected with an oseltamivir-resistant 2009 H1N1 virus and were too young to inhale zanamivir or were on ventilators and could not be given zanamivir because this drug cannot be used in intubated patients.

The problem of inadequate supplies of oseltamivir suspension was partially overcome by pharmacies breaking open the capsules and mixing the contents with a liquid sweetener. Reformulating oseltamivir into a suspension worked for children > 1 year of age, but this was not adequate for those < 12 months of age because of the small doses required by infants. To help alleviate this problem some of the limited supplies of oseltamivir pediatric suspension were released from the federal Strategic National Stockpile in October 2009 to the states and in turn to local health departments. The decision to use this limited supply of pediatric suspension in these infants was made because oseltamivir was the only drug approved for use in infants < 12 months of age and this age group represented the population at highest risk for hospitalization due to the 2009 H1N1 virus.

During the pandemic, the use of oseltamivir was approved for use in children < 1 year of age via the Emergency Use Authorization issued by the Food and Drug Administration. Previously the Food and Drug Administration label had indicated that this drug was contraindicated in this age group. The Emergency Use Authorization allows access to drugs that have not yet been licensed by the Food and Drug Administration or not been approved for a specific age group or indication. An Emergency Use Authorization is issued only if there is an emergency situation such as a pandemic and the drug being approved is believed to likely have efficacy based on the scientific evidence that is available at that point. How these drugs are to be used is set out in the Emergency Use Authorization and the use of the drug does not require informed consent by the patient or approval by an institutional review board (IRB). An Emergency Use Authorization was also issued for intravenous peramivir, a drug that had not been previously licensed by the Food and Drug Administration, but was needed for 2009 H1N1-infected hospitalized patients who could not take oral medications.

The scarcity of the liquid formulation led some pharmacies to markedly increase the price of the liquid preparation of oseltamivir. A *USA Today* phone survey of > 100 pharmacies found a range in pricing from $43 to $130. The increased pricing led Attorney Generals in a number of states, including Connecticut and Mississippi, to initiate investigations into price gouging.[85]

Many authorities remained concerned that overuse of oseltamivir would lead to increased levels of resistance. Therefore, in most countries, the use of oseltamivir and zanamivir for treatment or prophylaxis were limited to those at high risk of complications. However, Norway and a few other countries took the opposite approach and made oseltamivir available without the need for a prescription. The rationale for doing so was to decrease the stress caused by the pandemic on their healthcare system. The experience in other countries where this antiviral drug was readily available suggested that making this drug readily available to the public reduced the number of outpatient visits to physician offices and emergency departments. Additionally, preliminary data suggested that early use of oseltamivir was associated with a lower incidence of severe disease due to the 2009 H1N1 virus. While using this drug over the counter might facilitate the emergence of antiviral drug resistance, <100 virus isolates with the 274/275Y mutation that conferred resistance had been reported at that time despite the widespread use of this drug. Two small clusters have been reported in the USA and UK in severely immunocompromised persons, but otherwise all isolates have been from unconnected individuals who had been on oseltamivir treatment or prophylaxis. Thus, viruses with this mutation did not appear to be easily transmissible between people.

5.1.3 *Prevention of Disease in the Healthcare Setting*

A KEY POINT: Decreasing the risk of nosocomial infection in the healthcare setting was also considered a very important part of this overall effort to prevent disease and a number of interventions were employed including the use of appropriate isolation of patients, personal protective equipment for patients and HCWs, restriction of visitation and the use of antivirals and vaccines. Some of the recommendations on how to use these interventions became quite controversial including the declarations by the USA Occupational Safety and Health Administration and CDC on the type of mask to be used and the decision by some medical centers to mandate that all HCWs get the seasonal and pandemic vaccines as a condition of their continuing employment.

The question of what was the best type of mask to use to protect HCWs from nosocomially acquired 2009 H1N1 virus infection became a hotly debated issue. Two recently published studies did not show a difference in protection between standard surgical-type masks and N95 respirator masks.[86,87]

N95 respirators must be fit tested before they are used by HCWs. Fit testing is a process by which trained personnel test the N95 respirator on individual HCWs to make sure there are no air leaks. Fitting HCWs with a N95 respirator placed a substantial burden on medical centers since the process takes 10–15 minutes per HCW (and sometimes much longer when fitting proved difficult for individual HCWs and in some cases an adequate fit could not be achieved) and needs to be done each time N95 respirators are purchased from a different company (different companies make different models of N95 respirators and having to redo this process for each model was a frequent occurrence due to ongoing shortages of the N95 respirators). The WHO and Society for Healthcare Epidemiology of America recommended the use of surgical masks for most patients, but the CDC and the Occupational Safety and Health Administration were recommending N95 fitted respirator masks.[57,88]

On October 14, the CDC issued further guidance on infection control measures for the 2009 H1N1 virus in the healthcare setting. This guidance reiterated earlier CDC recommendations for the use of respiratory protection that is at least as protective as a fit-tested disposable N95 respirator for HCWs who are in close contact with patients with suspected or confirmed 2009 H1N1 influenza. The North Carolina Department of Labor Occupational Safety and Health Division indicated that they would use the Occupational Safety and Health Administration's and the CDC's guidance on respiratory protection against the 2009 H1N1 virus as the regulatory standard when determining whether to issue citations.

Since these N95 respirators were in short supply, the Occupational Safety and Health Administration had to allow and provide guidance on the re-use of these respirators. Re-use of disposable N95 respirators, where the respirator is removed and re-donned between patient encounters, can result in a risk of contact transmission by touching a contaminated surface of the respirator and subsequently touching the mucous membranes of the face. The precise balance between risk of contact transmission and benefit of re-use associated with this strategy is unknown, although the risk can be minimized if HCWs perform hand hygiene every time before and after touching the respirator. The Occupational Safety and Health Administration recommended extended use (i.e., wearing over multiple encounters while minimizing touching, removing or re-donning between encounters) over re-use because it involved less touching of the respirator and face. The Occupational Safety and Health Administration also recommended that consultation with a medical center's infection control experts should be sought in making decisions regarding the most appropriate and feasible personal protective equipment to protect workers from influenza if N95 respirator shortages occur. If re-use was chosen as a strategy to increase availability of respiratory protection, the Occupational Safety and Health Administration recommended the following to minimize risk of transmission:

- Discard disposable N95 respirators following aerosol-generating procedures.
- Discard disposable N95 respirators contaminated with blood, respiratory or nasal secretions, or other bodily fluids from patients.
- Disposable respirators must only be used and re-used by a single wearer.
- Do not re-use a disposable respirator that is obviously contaminated, damaged or hard to breathe through.
- Consider use of a face shield over a disposable N95 respirator to prevent surface contamination.
- Store the respirator in a clean, breathable container such as a paper bag between uses.
- Avoid touching the inside of the respirator.
- Wearer should perform hand hygiene with soap and water or an alcohol-based hand sanitizer before and after touching a used respirator.

These recommendations were problematic in that they were more complex and time consuming than those associated with use of standard masks. Furthermore, HCWs did not like having to wear the respirators continuously (i.e., extended use). A previous study had shown that ≤30% HCWs were willing to wear these devices throughout an entire shift. The reasons cited include, but are not limited to, difficulty communicating with others and discomfort.[89] Most HCWs chose to re-use these respirators; however, the recommendation to avoid touching the inside of the respirator proved difficult and very few HCWs wore face shields.

The CDC and Occupational Safety and Health Administration acknowledged that shortages of N95 respirators were occurring. The guidance recommended prioritization of respiratory protection during respirator shortages. When prioritization was necessary, standard masks were recommended for employees at lower risk of exposure to the 2009 H1N1 virus or at less risk of developing severe infection. The guidance also indicated that facilities should maintain a reserve of N95 respirators sufficient to meet the estimated needs for performing aerosol-generating procedures and for managing patients with diseases other than influenza that require respiratory protection until supplies were replenished. Unfortunately, orders for additional N95 respirators were backordered for up to nine months and therefore most medical facilities could only count on being able to use N95 respirators already on site. Furthermore, the shortages of N95 respirators forced medical centers to purchase different makes, models or styles of respirators from what they had been using. This proved to be very difficult to implement due to the additional manpower, time and financial costs involved in refitting a large number of HCWs. The Occupational Safety and Health Administration did indicate that employers would be considered to be in compliance if they showed a good-faith effort had been made to acquire N95 respirators. The Society for Healthcare Epidemiology of America issued a statement reiterating its July 2009 position that opposed the CDC's and Occupational Safety and Health Administration's position that healthcare facilities should prioritize use of N95 fit-tested respirators over the standard masks (http://docs.google.com/viewer?a=v&q=cache:r8Tmb7web8YJ:www.shea-online.org/Assets/files/policy/061209_H1N1. The Society's position continued to be that N95 respirators should be reserved only for procedures associated with a higher risk of aerosolization of the virus, and that the main emphasis for protecting HCWs should be on the use of the pandemic and seasonal influenza vaccines.

The fact that the WHO and Society for Healthcare Epidemiology of America disagreed with the CDC and Occupational Safety and Health Administration about the adequacy of using standard masks was a major problem. The fact that the WHO, CDC and Society for Healthcare Epidemiology of America make recommendations, while the Occupational Safety and Health Administration can mandate a policy meant that medical centers actually were taking a regulatory compliance risk if they did not follow the Occupational Safety and Health Administration's policy. After the second wave of the pandemic was over in the USA, the Occupational Safety and Health Administration fined a number of hospitals for not using N95 masks and some of these hospitals have initiated appeals that are currently in process.

5.1.3.1 *Pregnant HCWs*

The epidemiologic data indicated that pregnant women were at particularly high risk for severe disease if they were infected with the 2009 H1N1 virus. The issue of what to do to help protect pregnant HCWs from getting infected while still maintaining adequate workforce capacity was of great importance, but there was no national consensus on how this could be achieved. Women HCWs often delay becoming pregnant until they are out of school and working. A decision not to allow pregnant HCWs to have contact with patients would have a substantial impact on the ability of medical centers to provide high-quality care to patients. Most medical centers provided HCWs with the appropriate information and education about the risk of the 2009 H1N1 virus to pregnant women and what they could do to decrease the risk at work and home (e.g., good hygiene, appropriate use of personal protective equipment, immunization when the vaccine became available, etc.) and then allowed each pregnant HCW to decide if they wanted to care only for those patients who were not suspected or proven to have 2009 H1N1 infection. Many pregnant

HCWs opted for this alternative and for the most part this did not prove to be disruptive in taking care of patients.

5.1.3.2 *Vaccination of HCWs*

Immunization of HCWs provides the most effective tool available to prevent them from getting influenza and also prevents HCWs from infecting their patients. Despite extensive educational efforts over many years, only ~45% of HCWs annually receive influenza vaccine. Based on the potential impact of the 2009 pandemic, the Association for Professionals in Infection Control and Epidemiology, the Infectious Diseases Society of America, the American College of Physicians and the National Society for Patient Safety urged healthcare institutions to require annual influenza vaccines for all employees with direct patient contact, and in 2009, to also require the pandemic vaccine.[58] The Association for Professionals in Infection Control and Epidemiology position paper "Influenza Immunization of Healthcare Personnel" noted that the current rate of HCW immunizations against influenza is appallingly low and must not be tolerated. The Association further stated that it was time for hospitals to require influenza shots and hold employees accountable for declining the vaccine. The Association noted that not doing so could cause medical centers a double problem of increased illness and absenteeism among staff, coupled with overcrowded facilities that often occur due to the increased numbers of patients hospitalized during influenza season.[88] The increase in the number of HCWs that were absent from work at Wake Forest University Baptist Medical Center during the second wave of the pandemic is shown in Fig. 26.

Wake Forest University Baptist Medical Center had worked for many years to increase the number of HCWs that received the seasonal influenza vaccine. Various methods were utilized including education sessions about the reasons to get vaccinated, providing the vaccine at no cost, vaccinating HCWs on the units where they worked, and requiring signed declination of those who refused to be vaccinated. While these efforts increased the vaccination rate at ~25% of HCWs were still not receiving influenza vaccine. Based on the potential impact of the second wave of the pandemic

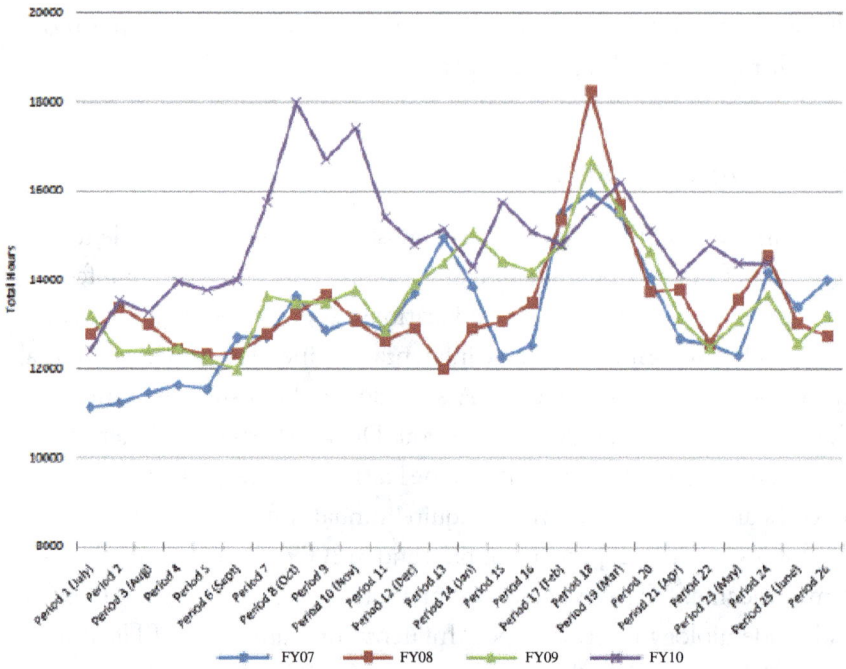

Fig. 26. The impact of the pandemic on the number of hospital HCWs at Wake Forest University Baptist Medical Center that were absent from work during the fiscal years (FY) 2007, 2008, 2009 and 2010 (at Wake Forest University Baptist Medical Center the fiscal year runs from July 1–June 30).

on the ability to provide care for a large number of patients if increased numbers of employees were out sick due to seasonal or pandemic influenza, the medical center leadership decided to require that all HCWs receive both the seasonal and pandemic vaccines in the 2009–2010 season and the seasonal vaccine annually thereafter as a condition for continued employment. Wake Forest University Baptist Medical Center issued the following policy statement on influenza vaccination on September 24, 2009:

Employee Influenza Immunization Policy

It is the policy and the deep commitment of Wake Forest University Baptist Medical Center to protect our patients, employees, students, trainees, volunteers and the community as a whole from influenza infection. Influenza vaccination is essential to protect the health and safety of all and is a critical tool that will help us meet the significant challenges of seasonal and H1N1 influenza that lie ahead.

Wake Forest University Baptist Medical Center has ratified a new policy requiring influenza immunization for all faculty, regular and contract staff, students, post-doctoral trainees and volunteers within the Medical Center and its subsidiaries. The new policy applies both to seasonal and H1N1 influenza vaccines and was implemented on September 23.

Leaders from Human Resources, Employee Health Services and Infectious Diseases have compiled an extensive question and answer document that includes our influenza immunization program, common questions and concerns about influenza vaccinations, exemptions, and questions about H1N1.

Wake Forest University Baptist Medical Center has for many years benefited from high voluntary compliance with seasonal influenza vaccination, so, for most of us, getting our influenza shots will simply be business as usual. We recognize, however, that some employees will require exemptions. Conditions that may be considered for exemption and workplace requirements for those employees who cannot be vaccinated are detailed in the accompanying intranet links. Please email any questions to askus@wfubmc.edu.

Seasonal influenza shots will be available on the main Wake Forest Baptist campus starting today, Thursday, Sept. 24, at Employee Health Services and later at various locations across the Medical Center and off-site. Please complete and print the *online consent form*, then bring it with you when you come for your vaccine. (Subsidiaries will provide vaccine communications and schedules to their employee communities.)

We anticipate the first deliveries of limited quantities of H1N1 vaccine in early October. Employee groups identified as first priority recipients will be alerted by email. You will be updated about the vaccine as information becomes available.

In this rapidly changing health environment, it is important for you to refer often to the intranet H1N1 site for the latest information and clinical guidance for H1N1, as well as to the intranet seasonal influenza site for updates on vaccine sites and general influenza information.

We anticipate an extremely challenging influenza season ahead, and we all must do our part to ensure our readiness and ability to deliver patient care under demanding circumstances. We greatly appreciate your cooperation and compliance with the new influenza vaccine mandate. As always, thank you for all that you do to ensure that we provide the best possible care to our patients and the safest environment for our employees.

The week prior to sending out this memo, several town hall meetings were held where faculty and staff were invited to hear a short presentation about the pandemic and the rationale for this new mandatory vaccine policy. At each town hall meeting, a substantial amount of time was allotted for questions and comments. Based in part on the discussions at these meetings, the following Questions and Answers document was developed and sent along with the new mandatory vaccine policy to every HCW:

Employee Influenza Immunization Policy
Questions and Answers

These questions and answers below apply to both seasonal and pandemic influenza and to their respective vaccines. There is also a section near the end of this document specifically addressing just H1N1.

Why is Wake Forest University Baptist Medical Center requiring employees to receive the influenza vaccine?

Our goal is to do everything possible to protect the safety of our patients, our employees and their families, and our community. Influenza vaccination is a critical part of protecting everyone from the spread of illness.

My job does not involve direct patient contact. Why am I required to get vaccinated?

Everyone who is not vaccinated is at risk of contracting and spreading the influenza to others. Our goal is to prevent influenza among our patient and employee populations and any unvaccinated employees compromise patient and employee safety.

Does the Employee Influenza Immunization Policy apply to volunteers and contract staff?

Yes. The policy applies to all Wake Forest University Baptist Medical Center employees, which include faculty, full-time, part-time, and PRN staff, House Officers, contract staff, and volunteers of Wake Forest University Baptist Medical Center.

Are other hospitals requiring their employees to be vaccinated?

Yes. A number of healthcare organizations across our region and the country are implementing policies similar to ours for the protection of their patients and employees.

What happens if I refuse to be vaccinated?

Any employee who fails to comply with the requirements of the Employee Influenza Immunization Policy will become ineligible to work at Wake Forest University Baptist Medical Center. Anyone in any of the other groups listed above who fails to comply as well will become ineligible to be on any Wake

Forest University Baptist Medical Center campus or work with its patients, personnel, facilities, or other resources.

Questions about the Employee Influenza Immunization Program

What is the Employee Influenza Immunization Program?

Each year, Employee Health Services (EHS) coordinates an influenza vaccination campaign. EHS establishes the dates for the campaign and coordinates vaccination schedules to ensure that all employees are able to receive their vaccine while at work. Wake Forest University Baptist Medical Center provides the vaccine free of charge to all Medical Center employees.

When will the influenza vaccine be available?

This year's Influenza Immunization Program is scheduled to begin on September 24th.

What is the deadline for getting the vaccine?

All employees must be either vaccinated or granted an exemption within 30 days of being offered the vaccine.

Where do I go to get my influenza shot?

Employee Health Services (EHS) coordinates both vaccination schedules and locations throughout the Medical Center. Additionally, unit-based vaccinators again will help administer the vaccine. You may get your vaccination at EHS or check with your manager to see where vaccinations will be provided near your work area. This information will also be displayed at EHS and on the EHS Flu web page.

I work nights and weekends. How will I get my vaccination?

EHS ensures that the vaccination schedule covers all work shifts. Please watch for communications regarding vaccination schedules or speak to your manager. Also, refer to the question above.

I got vaccinated at my doctor's office (or other location). What do I need to do?

You must provide proof of immunization to EHS. Acceptable forms of proof are a doctor's note or immunization record.

Can my family members come to Wake Forest University Baptist Medical Center for a free vaccination?

EHS schedules Family Flu Night events at the Medical Center, at which family members can receive the seasonal influenza vaccine at a cost of $20 per person. Family Flu Nights are contingent upon availability of sufficient influenza vaccine to cover all employees first.

Common Questions, Concerns, and Myths about Influenza Vaccinations

Can I get the influenza vaccine if I am pregnant or breastfeeding?

Yes. According to the CDC, *pregnant women and breastfeeding mothers* are among those who *should be vaccinated*. Pregnant women are at high risk of complications from the influenza if they become ill during their pregnancy and breastfeeding mothers should be vaccinated to avoid passing the influenza to their babies.

What are the side effects of the influenza vaccine?

The side effects of the vaccine are minimal and most people are unaffected. Some experience a mildly sore arm for a short time, a mild fever and/or minor aches that last about 24 hours. There is also a possible, albeit rare, association with Guillain-Barre syndrome (GBS).

I got the influenza from the influenza shot last time.

Influenza vaccines *cannot* cause the influenza. If you became ill with the influenza after receiving the influenza vaccine, it is most likely that you either contracted it before you received the shot or contracted a virus for which the vaccine did not provide protection.

I don't consider the influenza to be dangerous, so I don't need influenza shot.

Influenza can have serious medical complications leading to more than 200,000 hospitalizations and 36,000 deaths in the USA each year. Vaccination is the best protection against the influenza.

I don't think influenza vaccines really work.

The ability of vaccines to protect depends upon people's age and health status, as well as how well matched the vaccine is to the virus strains that are going around. However, when vaccines are well matched, they can reduce the changes of getting the influenza by nearly 90 percent.

I am afraid of shots.

All the nurse vaccinators are quite experienced in giving injections, minimizing the discomfort. For those who do not want an injection, nasal sprays are available for the seasonal vaccine and also the pandemic vaccine for healthy adults <50 years of age.

Exemptions from the Influenza Immunization Policy

Can I request to be exempt from the immunization policy?

Exemptions may be granted for certain medical conditions or religious beliefs.

What is required for a medical exemption?

Medical exemptions may be granted to employees with a documented severe allergy to eggs or latex or a history of GBS. To request a medical exemption, you must provide proof of a qualifying medical condition to EHS within thirty days of the start of the Influenza Immunization Program (this year, within thirty days of September 24).

How do I request a religious exemption?

To request a religious exemption, you must provide a written request to EHS within thirty days of the start of the influenza immunization program (this year, within thirty days of September 24). Your written request should clearly explain why the immunization is contrary to your religious beliefs.

How will I know if my exemption has been granted?

Your request for exemption will be reviewed and you will receive a written response within five business days of presenting your request to EHS. In some cases, EHS may need to request additional information from you, in which case, you will receive a written response to your request within five business days of providing all requested information.

If I am granted an exemption, will I be allowed to perform my regular job duties?

You will be permitted to perform your regular work duties. However, you will be required to wear a surgical or isolation mask in all patient care areas while at work during the influenza season.

Questions Specific to the H1N1 Vaccine

Does the Wake Forest University Baptist Medical Center Influenza Immunization Policy apply to the H1N1 vaccine?

Yes. The policy will be a standing policy for the seasonal influenza vaccine but may also be applied to influenza viruses for which the seasonal influenza vaccine does not provide protection.

Will the H1N1 vaccine be separate from the regular seasonal vaccine?

Yes, this year's seasonal influenza vaccine does not provide protection against the pandemic H1N1 influenza A virus. A separate vaccine has been developed for the virus.

When will the H1N1 vaccine be available?

We anticipate that we will begin receiving the H1N1 vaccine around the middle of October. However, we do not yet know the quantity that we will be able to obtain or the rate at which we will receive it over time.

Will all employees be required to get the H1N1 vaccine?

It is unlikely that enough vaccine will initially be available to immunize all Medical Center employees against the H1N1 influenza. Criteria will be established for the order in which employees will receive the H1N1 vaccine with priority given to employees who provide direct, hands-on patient care or have a high risk of exposure to patients with the influenza. Employees who are identified to receive the vaccine will be required to be immunized.

Has the H1N1 vaccine been clinically tested and is it safe?

We have every reason to believe it will be safe — this vaccine will be made using the same processes and facilities that are used to make the currently licensed seasonal influenza vaccines. The US Food and Drug Administration announced the week of September 14th that it has approved vaccines against the 2009 H1N1 virus made by four manufacturing companies. For more information see http://www.cdc.gov/h1n1flu/.

If I have already had the H1N1 influenza, do I still need to be vaccinated?

If you were ill with a fever and respiratory symptoms AFTER August 1, 2009 AND TESTED POSITIVE FOR INFLUENZA by a documented rapid test or PCR, vaccination is NOT necessary. Otherwise vaccination is required, as other viruses besides influenza could have been responsible for the illness.

The prioritization scheme that was devised for HCWs at Wake Forest University Baptist Medical Center was based on consideration of which HCWs were at most risk of being exposed to patients with disease due to the 2009 H1N1 virus and also who was at most risk of developing severe disease if they did become infected. Additionally, LAIV was prioritized for those HCW groupings that were likely to have a large number of healthy adults <50 years of age (the upper age limit of the Food and Drug Administration label for LAIV). The scheme is noted below in descending order of priority:

(1) TIV for those who worked in the bone marrow and solid organ transplant units.
(2) TIV or LAIV for those working in the emergency department or obstetrical unit.

(3) LAIV for all healthy housestaff, medical students and physician assistants except for those who would be in the bone marrow transplant unit within several weeks of receiving the vaccine.
(4) TIV or LAIV for those working in pediatric inpatient or outpatient sites.
(5) TIV or LAIV for self-identified high-risk employees.
(6) TIV or LAIV for those working in the adult critical care and oncology units.
(7) TIV or LAIV for those working in adult inpatient or outpatient sites.

5.1.3.3 *Rumors and myths appearing on the internet once the mandatory vaccine policy was announced*

As soon as some of the medical centers announced that they were going to require all HCWs to be vaccinated, various rumors and myths started to appear about the 2009 pandemic vaccine. Some of these included that (see text in italics for why these rumors and myths were incorrect):

- The vaccine to be used in the USA contained adjuvants and additives not found in the seasonal influenza vaccine. *Although many countries decided to use adjuvanted H1N1 vaccine, only non-adjuvanted vaccine was used in the USA.*
- One of the companies had produced a vaccine containing 40 times the usual amount of thimerosal found in some of the seasonal influenza vaccines. *This and similar accusations about thimerosal were unfounded, but concerns about thimerosal continued to occur despite the fact that there is overwhelming scientific evidence that thimerosal does not cause autism.*
- The first day the pandemic vaccine became available, a child developed GBS due to the vaccine. *It is biologically impossible for GBS to occur the day the vaccine was given since GBS is caused by auto-antibodies that are formed weeks after the person is exposed to the causative agent.*

5.1.3.4 *Impact of the mandatory influenza vaccine policy on Wake Forest University Baptist Medical Center HCW immunization rates*

A total of 14,018 Medical Center faculty, staff, students and volunteers were required to receive the pandemic and seasonal influenza vaccines during the 2009–2010 season. The Medical Center achieved over 99% compliance with mandatory immunization for pandemic influenza with 13,985 employees and volunteers receiving the vaccine on-site, providing proof of outside immunization, or requesting exemption based on medical contraindications or religious beliefs. Medical exemptions were requested by 171 people, 138 of which were granted. Religious exemptions were requested by 87 people and approved for 68. Ten volunteers and nine employees elected to leave the Medical Center, rather than to comply with the immunization policy.

Due to periodic shortages of seasonal vaccine during most of the influenza season, the Medical Center was not able to fully implement the mandatory vaccination policy for seasonal influenza. Despite these shortages, 80% of the HCWs were immunized for seasonal influenza with 11,175 employees and volunteers receiving the vaccine on-site, providing proof of outside immunization, or requesting exemption.

The state of New York tried to mandate that the pandemic and seasonal influenza vaccines be required of all HCWs who have contact with patients in hospitals and other specified settings. Additionally, a substantial number of individual hospitals across the country developed similar policies. In some cases, the policy of requiring HCWs to get the influenza vaccine was challenged by unions or individual HCWs in the courts. While in some cases temporary restraining orders were issued (e.g., the statewide requirement in New York), in most instances the hospitals prevailed.[90] Compared to those employers who neither required nor recommended influenza vaccination for their employees, those who required influenza seasonal and 2009 H1N1 influenza vaccination had an almost twofold and eightfold higher rate of vaccination, respectively.[91]

5.1.4 *Hospital Visitation Restrictions*

Most medical centers already had established signage and screening procedures in place during seasonal influenza to help ensure that friends and relatives of patients were not entering patient rooms if they had signs and symptoms of influenza. During the 2009 pandemic, many medical centers instituted more restrictive visitation policies. Wake Forest University Baptist Medical Center joined with a number of other hospitals in the region to limit hospital visitation to people $\geq$18 years of age since those who were younger had the greatest incidence of infection and were more likely to transmit disease to patients and HCWs. Exceptions to this policy were approved on a case by case basis by the patient's physician when the benefit of the visitation was thought to outweigh the risk of transmission of infection. Adult visitors continued to be screened by unit staff for fever and respiratory symptoms prior to entering the patient's room.

Another particularly difficult infection control issue concerned what to do with pregnant women with suspected or confirmed 2009 H1N1 infection and their newborns. CDC guidelines[92] recommended that the mother be separated from their infant and not be allowed to visit the baby in the nursery or have the newborn room in until the mother was no longer contagious (usually considered to be 24 hours after their fever had abated without the use of antipyretics). Mothers who were allowed to go home while still having influenza-like illness symptoms were recommended to have someone else take care of the infant until they were no longer contagious. Due to the substantial increased risk that a young infant infected with the 2009 H1N1 virus would require hospitalization, most mothers were willing to abide by these recommendations.

5.2 The Possibility of a Third Pandemic Wave Occurring

As the second wave of the pandemic was receding in the Northern Hemisphere, the Southern Hemisphere was actively preparing for the start of their second wave. While most experts believed that a second wave would occur in both regions, many experts also believed that a third wave was likely to occur, most likely sometime in 2010 in the Northern Hemisphere. Margaret Chan, Director-General of the WHO, noted at the end of 2009 that another year or more of monitoring the pandemic was needed to determine whether the pandemic had peaked. She emphasized that a mutation of the 2009 pandemic virus to a more severe form was still possible.

In the USA the concern about a third wave was heightened by the fact that CDC influenza-like illness surveillance data suggested that only ~47 million people (15%) in the USA had been infected with the 2009 H1N1 virus while in previous pandemics about 30% of the population had developed influenza-like illness. While some of the population had also been vaccinated, the majority of the world's population still remained at risk for developing disease. There was also a concern that seasonal influenza viruses would occur during the first quarter of 2010. At the time of publication of this book a third wave had not yet occurred anywhere in the world.

References

65. The 2009 pandemic H1N1 influenza and indigenous populations of the Americas and the Pacific. (2009) *Eurosurveillance* **14** (October 22).
66. Centers for Disease Control and Prevention (CDC). (2009) Deaths related to 2009 pandemic influenza A (H1N1) among American Indian/Alaska Natives — 12 states, 2009. MMWR **58**: 1341–1344.
67. Kilander A, Rykkvin R, Dudman SG, Hunges O. (2010) Observed association between the HA1 mutation D222G in the 2009 pandemic influenza A(H1N1) virus and severe clinical outcomes, Norway 2009–2010. *Eurosurveillance* **15**:pii=19498.
68. Centers for Disease Control and Prevention (CDC). 2009 H1N1 Flu: International Situation Update [http://www.cdc.gov/h1n1flu/updates/international, accessed January 22, 2010].
69. Trust for America's Health. (2009) H1N1 Challenges Ahead, October, 1–38 [www.healthyamericans.org].
70. Centers for Disease Control and Prevention CDC. CDC Estimates of 2009 H1N1 Influenza Cases, Hospitalizations and Deaths in the United States,

April–December 2009 [http://www.cdc.gov/h1n1flu/estimates_2009_h1n1.htm, accessed January 15, 2010].

71. Centers for Disease Control and Prevention (CDC). U.S. Influenza-Associated Pediatric Mortality [http://www.cdc.gov/h1n1flu/updates/us/#pedh1n1cares, accessed January 29, 2010].

72. Viboud C, Miller M, Olson D *et al.* (2009) Preliminary estimates of mortality and years of life lost associated with the 2009 A/H1N1 pandemic in the US and comparison with past influenza seasons. *PLOS Currents* [http://knol.google.com/k/cecile-viboud/preliminary-estimates-of-mortality-and/35hpbywfdwl4n/8?collectionId=28qm4w0q65e4w.1&position=2#].

73. Australia and New Zealand Extracorporeal Membrane Oxygenation (ANZ ECMO) Influenza Investigators, Davies A, Jones D, Bailey M *et al.* (2009) Extracorporeal membrane oxygenation for 2009 influenza A(H1N1) acute respiratory distress syndrome. *JAMA* **302**: 1888–1895.

74. Writing Committee of the WHO Consultation on Clinical Aspects of Pandemic (H1N1) Influenza. (2010) Clinical aspects of pandemic 2009 influenza A (H1N1) virus infection. *N Engl J Med* **362**: 1708–1719.

75. Plennevaux E, Sheldon E, Blatter M *et al.* (2010) Immune response after a single vaccination against 2009 influenza A H1N1 in United States: A preliminary report of two randomized controlled phase 2 trials. *Lancet* **375**: 41–48.

76. Fiore AE, Neuzil KM. (2010) 2009 influenza A (H1N1) monovalent vaccines for children. *JAMA* **303**: 73–74.

77. Skowronski DM, De Serres G, Crowcroft NS *et al.* (2010) Association between the 2008–09 seasonal influenza vaccine and pandemic H1N1 illness during spring–summer 2009: Four observational studies from Canada. *PLoS Med* **7**: e1000258 [doi:10.1371/journal.pmed.1000258].

78. Viboud C, Simonsen L. (2010) Does seasonal influenza vaccination increase the risk of illness with the 2009 A/H1N1 pandemic virus? *PLoS Med* **7**: e1000259.

79. Centers for Disease Control and Prevention (CDC). (2010) Interim results: State-specific influenza A (H1N1) 2009 monovalent vaccination coverage — United States, October 2009–January 2010. *MMWR* **59**: 363–368.

80. Low turnout at city clinics for free swine flu vaccine. (2009) National Network Immunization Newsbrief, November 12.

81. Swine flu vaccines hijacked in Milwaukee. (2009) PRESS TV, November 7.

82. Centers for Disease Control and Prevention (CDC). (2010) Interim results: Influenza A (H1N1) 2009 monovalent vaccination coverage — United States, October–December 2009. *MMWR* **59**: 44–48.

83. Millions of H1N1 vaccine doses may have to be discarded. (2010) *The Washington Post*, April 1 [http://www.washingtonpost.com/wp-dyn/content/article/2010/03/31/AR2010033104201.html].

84. Centers for Disease Control and Prevention (CDC). Questions and answers. Vaccine selection for the 2010–2011 influenza season [http://www.cdc.gov/flu/about/qa/1011_ vac_selection.htm, updated February 23, 2010].

85. Young A. (2009) Prices for H1N1 drug Tamiflu vary widely for same dose. *USA Today*, November 17 [www.usatoday.com/news/health/2009-11-17-swine-flu-drug-prices_N.htm].

86. Loeb M, Dafoe N, Mahony J et al. (2009) Surgical mask vs N95 respirator for preventing influenza among health care workers: A randomized trial. *JAMA* **302**: 1865–1871.

87. Ang B, Poh BF, Win MK, Chow A. (2010) Surgical masks for protection of health care personnel against pandemic novel swine-origin influenza A (H1N1) — 2009: Results from an observational study. *Clin Infect Dis* **50**: 1011–1014.

88. Association for Professionals in Infection Control and Epidemiology. (2008) Position Paper: Influenza immunization of healthcare personnel [http://www.apic.org/Content/NavigationMenu/PracticeGuidance/HealthcareWorkers-InfectionPrevention/Healthcare_Worker_R.htm].

89. Shine KI, Rogers B, Goldfrank LR. (2009) Novel H1N1 influenza and respiratory protection for health care workers. *N Engl J Med* **361**: 1823–1825.

90. Parmet WE. (2010) Pandemic vaccines — The legal landscape. *N Engl J Med* **362**: 1949–1952.

91. Centers for Disease Control and Prevention (CDC). (2010) Interim results: Influenza A (H1N1) 2009 monovalent and seasonal influenza vaccination coverage among health-care personnel — United States, August 2009–January 2010. *MMWR* **59**: 357–362.

92. Centers for Disease Control and Prevention (CDC). Updated interim recommendations for obstetric care providers related to use of antiviral medications in the treatment and prevention of influenza for the 2009–2010 season. [http:// www.cdc.gov/H1N1flu/pregnancy/antiviral_messages.htm, updated December 29, 2009].

Chapter 6

The Effectiveness of Pandemic Planning in Mitigating Disease

"By three methods we may learn wisdom: First, by reflection, which is noblest; second, by imitation, which is easiest; and third by experience, which is the bitterest."

Confucius

6.1 Analysis of the Effectiveness of the USA Pandemic Strategy

6.1.1 *Stop, Slow, or Otherwise Limit the Spread of a Pandemic into the United States*

> A KEY POINT: While this chapter discusses the successes and failures of the USA pandemic planning strategy, many of these lessons are applicable to other countries that had created similar plans. Of all the specific goals that were in the 2005 USA pandemic plan, the first goal that involved plans to stop, slow or limit the spread of the 2009 H1N1 virus into the USA was felt by those who devised the Strategy to be the most difficult to achieve. Their concern proved to be correct.

Many emerging infectious disease events have occurred due to passage of microbes from animals to humans. During the past 60 years, >65% of emerging infections have emerged from zoonotic sources.[93] Countries are

145

frequently not medically prepared to deal with these emerging diseases, as was the case with HIV/AIDS and variant Creutzfeldt–Jakob disease (the human form of "mad cow disease"). The severity of illness due to an emerging infection is often unpredictable and widely variable. For example, the 1918 influenza pandemic was caused by a particularly virulent strain of H1N1 virus that killed many millions of people worldwide, while the 1968 pandemic caused by a new H3N2 virus caused far fewer deaths.

Given the rapid speed of influenza virus transmission and the susceptibility of most, if not all, people, an outbreak of pandemic influenza anywhere poses a risk to populations everywhere. Stopping an outbreak had been achieved with other viral diseases (e.g., the outbreak of severe acute respiratory syndrome [SARS] that was caused by a new coronavirus). However, for a variety of reasons, including the high attack rate and short incubation periods associated with influenza, the possibility that an influenza pandemic could be contained outside the USA was felt by many experts to be unlikely, since many countries lacked the necessary resources, infrastructure or expertise to detect and respond to influenza outbreaks independently. Additionally, coordinated international mechanisms to support effective global surveillance and response were also inadequate.

In response to this concern, the United States Agency for International Development (USAID) asked the Institute of Medicine and the National Research Council to provide advice on how to achieve a more sustainable global capacity for surveillance and response to emerging zoonotic diseases. A committee was convened to examine several infectious disease surveillance systems already in operation, identify effective systems, uncover gaps in efforts and recommend improvements toward the goal of an effective global disease surveillance system. The committee concluded that there is no single example, in the USA or elsewhere, of a well-functioning zoonotic disease surveillance system integrated across human and animal health sectors.[93]

The committee noted that the USA government is among the world leaders in disease surveillance and has a considerable stake in the emergence and spread of zoonotic diseases. They recommended that the USA lead a collaborative effort that includes other countries, the private sector and nongovernmental organizations to coordinate a global, integrated and sustainable zoonotic disease surveillance system. Strategic approaches to strengthen surveillance and response included:

- Working with researchers to develop science-based criteria to determine the magnitude and distribution of disease drivers.
- Immediately strengthening surveillance in human populations at high risk for zoonotic diseases (e.g., livestock and poultry workers) in countries where disease surveillance in animal populations is weak.
- Developing and strengthening surveillance systems in animal populations so that outbreaks are detected early in animal populations rather than discovered later through secondary human outbreaks, as was the case with the 2009 pandemic.
- Synchronizing and sharing surveillance information from both human and animal populations in an integrated system, in as close to real time as possible.
- Engaging science-based, nongovernmental organizations as valuable partners that provide the wide geographic reach and field expertise needed for more comprehensive surveillance and response activities.

These general recommendations and other more specific actions (e.g., eliminating incentives for disease concealment at the country and local levels and reducing the social and economic repercussions for early reporting) were only beginning to be implemented when the 2009 H1N1 virus caused the pandemic. Had these recommended actions been in place earlier, they might have been able to slow down the spread of the virus worldwide, but it is unlikely that they could have prevented the pandemic. Additionally, the lack of an available vaccine at the onset of a pandemic and the paucity of data indicating that antiviral agents could effectively be used in a mass prophylaxis campaign also contributed to the inability to prevent the 2009 pandemic. Additional research, preventive infrastructure and global collaboration are needed to potentially achieve this important goal.

The US public health system was receiving <2% of the total healthcare spending in the USA at the onset of the 2009 pandemic.[94] In December

2009, the Trust for America's Health and the Robert Wood Johnson Foundation released their seventh annual report *"Ready or Not? Protecting the Public's Health from Diseases, Disasters, and Bioterrorism"*.[95] This report noted that the 2009 pandemic had exposed serious underlying gaps in the nation's ability to respond to public health emergencies and the ongoing economic recession was further straining an already fragile public health system. The report found that 20 states scored 6 or less out of 10 on key indicators of public health emergency preparedness and that two-thirds of states scored 7 or less. These preparedness indicators were developed in consultation with leading public health experts based on data from publicly available sources and information provided by public officials. The scores of each state are noted below:*

- 3 out of 10: Montana
- 5 out of 10: Alaska, Arizona, Florida, Idaho, Maine, Washington
- 6 out of 10: Connecticut, Georgia, Illinois, Kansas, Louisiana, Nebraska, Nevada, New Jersey, New Mexico, Rhode Island, Utah, West Virginia, Wyoming
- 7 out of 10: Hawaii, Indiana, Iowa, Maryland, Massachusetts, Minnesota, Missouri, New Hampshire, South Dakota, Tennessee, Virginia
- 8 out of 10: Alabama, California, Colorado, District of Columbia, Kentucky, Michigan, Mississippi, Ohio, Oregon, Pennsylvania, South Carolina, Wisconsin
- 9 out of 10: Arkansas, Delaware, New York, North Carolina, North Dakota, Oklahoma, Texas, Vermont

*For the state-by-state scoring, states received one point for achieving an indicator or zero points if they did not achieve the indicator. Zero is the lowest possible overall score, 10 is the highest. The data for the indicators are from publicly available sources or were provided by public officials. A full list of all the indicators and scores as well as the entire report are available on the Robert Wood Johnson Foundation and Trust for America's Health websites at www.rwjf.org and www.healthyamericans.org, respectively.

The report did note that the investments made in pandemic and public health preparedness over the past several years had dramatically improved USA readiness for the H1N1 outbreak, but that decades of chronic underfunding of the public health infrastructure had resulted in core systems that were still not ready to deal with a pandemic. Some of the key infrastructure concerns were a lack of real-time coordinated disease surveillance and laboratory testing, outdated vaccine production capabilities, limited hospital surge capacity, and a shrinking public health workforce. In addition, >50% of the states experienced cuts to their public health funding, and federal preparedness funds had been cut by 27% since 2005, which put at risk the improvements made after the September 11, 2001 terrorist attack in New York City.

Some key findings from the report include:

- 27 states cut funding for public health from FY 2007–08 to 2008–09.
- 13 states have purchased less than 50% of their share of federally subsidized antiviral drugs to stockpile for use during a pandemic.
- 11 states and Washington, DC, reported not having enough laboratory staffing capacity to work five 12-hour days for six to eight weeks in response to an infectious disease outbreak, such as the 2009 H1N1 pandemic.

The report offered a series of recommendations for improving preparedness, including:

- Ensure Stable and Sufficient Funding: The 27% decrease in federal support for public health preparedness since FY 2005 must be restored, and funding stabilized at a sufficient level to support core activities and emergency planning. Increased funding must also be provided to modernize influenza vaccine production, improve vaccine and antiviral research and development, and fully support the Hospital Preparedness Program to increase surge capacity.
- Conduct an H1N1 After-Action Report and Update Preparedness Plans with Lessons Learned: Strengths and weaknesses of the 2009 H1N1 response should be evaluated and used to revise and strengthen federal, state and local preparedness planning, including assessing what

additional resources are needed to be sufficiently prepared. Identified gaps in core systems, including communications, surveillance and laboratories must be addressed. In addition, continued surge capacity concerns, including establishing crisis standards of care, must be addressed.

- Increase Accountability and Transparency: Federal and state health departments should regularly make updates on progress made on benchmarks and deliverables identified in the Pandemic and All-Hazards Preparedness Act available to the public so they can see how tax dollars are being used and how well protected their communities are from health threats.

- Improve Community Preparedness: Additional measures must be taken to reach out quickly and effectively to high-risk populations, including strengthening culturally competent communications around the safety of vaccines. Health disparities among low-income and racial/ethnic minorities, who are often at higher risk during emergencies, must also be addressed.

6.1.2 *Planning for the Prevention and Treatment of Disease*

A KEY POINT: A critical component of the Strategy's second goal was to have stockpiles of pre-pandemic vaccine in sufficient quantities to immunize 20 million people in the USA before the disease entered the country. This goal was in part designed with the avian influenza A (H5N1) virus in mind. However, unlike the H5N1 virus, the 2009 H1N1 virus was readily transmissible between people and therefore there was insufficient time to develop a stockpile of vaccine against the 2009 H1N1 virus. This goal was also not achieved because the first goal of slowing the spread of the pandemic virus was not successful. Furthermore, the federal government's projection, made in July 2009, of 120 million doses of pandemic vaccine available by October 2009 was too optimistic. By the end of October 2009 only ~28 million doses of pandemic vaccine were distributed for use and by then the second wave was well underway throughout the USA.

6.1.2.1 *Vaccines*

Protecting human health is the crux of pandemic preparedness, and the pillars of the **Strategy** reflect this point. Failure to protect human health would likely mean that the secondary goals of preserving societal function and mitigating the social and economic consequences of a pandemic would also fail. Consequently, the components of the **Strategy's** implementation plan and the projected allocation of resources to preparedness, surveillance and response activities all reflect the overarching imperative to reduce morbidity and mortality caused by a pandemic.

The features that make a virus likely to cause a pandemic include the fact that a large portion of the population has no immunity against the virus and the virus has the ability to easily transmit between people. Given these features, at the current time, the necessary tools to stop a highly contagious virus from rapidly spreading around the world are not available since the most effective way to prevent a pandemic requires a vaccine that contains the specific virus HA and NA proteins and the time to produce this vaccine is at least four months.

One approach that potentially could allow a pandemic vaccine to be produced in a time frame that allows the vaccine to be available before the virus becomes widespread is to develop technology that speeds up the process of making the currently available types of influenza vaccines (i.e., vaccines whose effectiveness is dependent on how closely the HA protein in the vaccine is matched to the HA of the circulating virus that is causing the pandemic). Until better tools are available to predict which new strain of influenza virus will cause a pandemic, preemptive production of a pandemic vaccine is unlikely to be a successful strategy (e.g., an avian H5N1 vaccine was made preemptively due to concerns that it would cause the next pandemic, but to date this avian pandemic has not occurred). The use of cell culture and recombinant technology will likely soon replace the egg-based systems as the predominant way of making influenza vaccines for worldwide use. In August 2010, the President's Council of Advisors on Science and Technology released a report containing recommendations to improve nation's vaccine response against pandemic influenza and other outbreaks (http://www.whitehouse.gov/administration/eop/ostp/pcast). While the recommendation in this report could speed up the time it takes to make the vaccine by several weeks to a month, these methods are still not likely to produce vaccines rapidly enough to prevent the worldwide spread of a pandemic virus. Additionally, some of the issues that plagued the production of the pandemic vaccine must also be solved, including difficulties in growing the vaccine strain, problems in rapidly getting the billions of doses of vaccine product into vials, the time it takes to obtain approval from the regulatory agencies in various countries, and distribution of vaccines to the world's population.

A potentially better approach to stopping the worldwide spread of a pandemic virus involves development of an influenza vaccine that contains a stable viral component(s) that offers the ability to protect against many different strains of influenza virus even as the virus evolves over time. This type of vaccine offers a number of potential advantages including that it could be used for both seasonal and pandemic influenza viruses, be produced prior to a pandemic and vaccine stocks could be rotated through storage facilities. A number of research groups have been working for years on developing this type of vaccine, and recently the National Institute of Health (NIH) announced that it has begun clinical trials in humans with a newly developed influenza vaccine that when tested in animals provided coverage against a broad array of influenza virus strains (http://www.nih.gov/news/health/jul2010/niaid-15.htm).

The USA government had established two primary vaccine goals: (1) establishment and maintenance of stockpiles of pre-pandemic vaccine adequate to immunize 20 million persons against influenza strains that present a pandemic threat; and (2) expansion of domestic influenza vaccine manufacturing surge capacity for the production of pandemic vaccines for the entire domestic population within six months of a pandemic declaration. The hope was to have these goals met by 2010, and a fair amount of progress had been made in these areas by the time of the onset of the 2009 pandemic. Even if enough vaccine could be made for the entire USA population in six months, the planning process that is used to develop a vaccine prioritization scheme for the sequential order in which various groups of people would get the vaccine as it became available would continue to be necessary. The US prioritization plan that was originally created in 2005, revised in 2008 and then again in 2009 was based on presumed (2005 and 2008) or actual (2009) epidemiologic data and revised estimates of vaccine availability (see Figs. 18 and 19 in Chapter 4 for the 2008 and 2009 prioritization schemes).[56] For the most part, the priority scheme that was recommended in July 2009 by the ACIP was followed by healthcare providers and enabled those who were most at risk to receive the pandemic vaccine first. However, only approximately one-third of those initially recommended to get the vaccine did so (see Table 18 in Chapter 5).

6.1.2.2 *Antivirals*

The federal government had established two primary goals for stockpiling existing antiviral medications: (1) establishment and maintenance of stockpiles adequate to treat 75 million persons, divided between Federal and State stockpiles; and (2) establishment and maintenance of a Federal stockpile of 6 million treatment courses reserved for containment efforts. In an effort to expand the medical armamentarium, the federal government also supports research projects to optimize dosing strategies for existing antiviral medications, identify novel drug targets and develop compounds that inhibit viral entry, replication and maturation. The stockpile goals for oseltamivir were met which proved very helpful since <1% of the 2009 H1N1 isolates were resistant to this drug and even those that were resistant remained sensitive to zanamivir. Peramivir, a neuraminidase inhibitor given intravenously, was approved by the FDA under the Emergency Use Authorization and was used, given to a small number of patients who could not take oseltamivir orally. None of the new classes of influenza drugs being developed to inhibit influenza by mechanisms different from the adamantanes and neuraminidase inhibitors were available for use during the 2009 pandemic, but the low percentage of 2009 H1N1 virus resistance to the neuraminidase inhibitors made this problem a relatively minor issue.

6.1.2.3 *Additional interventions to prevent infection*

Other steps used to try to stop or slow down the spread of a pandemic included isolation of infected patients, quarantine of exposed persons, screening at entry points into a country, closing of public facilities including schools, educational efforts on how to avoid infection including the use of masks and appropriate cough and cold hygiene. Quarantine at the level of families and individuals are a legitimate public health intervention for some infections (e.g., this method figured prominently in the public health response to SARS). However, the value of individual quarantine as a public health intervention is determined by the biology of the agent against which it is directed. Since influenza infection can be transmitted by persons who are not ill, and because viral shedding occurs prior to the onset of clinical illness, isolation of ill persons or exclusion from work of those who are ill could reduce, but would not prevent, transmission in public settings.

Early in the 2009 pandemic, the CDC issued an advisory that a school should be closed if there was a confirmed case of the 2009 H1N1 virus in a student in the school and all schools in a community should be closed if there were cases in two different schools. However, during the first wave of the 2009 pandemic, the overall rate of hospitalization and death was not severe and this recommendation was changed to have children stay home if they were ill, but not to close schools. The closing of schools for the 2009 summer recess appeared to slow the spread of the 2009 H1N1 virus, but soon after schools reopened, the second wave of the pandemic began.

The social and economic impact of school closures (e.g., parents having to stay home with well children) was substantial and these issues had to be weighed against the possible health benefits. Voluntary isolation of those who were ill until 24 hours after fever abated continued to be recommended, but quarantine measures were not employed given the widespread distribution of the virus. These types of interventions have substantial negative consequences, including the economic and the psychological impact associated with social isolation. Nevertheless, the value of school closings, isolating patients with pandemic influenza and quarantining their contacts is supported by recent modeling efforts and was done during the beginning of the outbreak before the pandemic was shown to be of only mild to moderate severity. Had the pandemic been more severe (e.g., similar to the 1918 pandemic), these additional interventions could have been justified.

6.1.3 *Impacting Disease Severity*

A KEY POINT: The 2009 pandemic again demonstrated that there could be a substantial difference between the overall mortality rate and the impact of the pandemic on various groups of people. The severity of the 2009 pandemic was relatively low for individuals who were previously healthy, but substantially higher for those with one or more underlying risk factors including those where the incidence had markedly increased since the last pandemic (e.g., diabetes). Additionally, the mean age of those dying was much younger than in most pandemics and this combination of increased numbers of people with high-risk conditions and a low median age of those who were dying meant that the total number of life years lost was substantial, making the impact of the pandemic much greater in those with underlying high-risk conditions.

The **Strategy** emphasized that the severity of a pandemic is not simply a function of the attack rate or transmissibility of the virus which appear to be relatively constant features of pandemics, but rather the ability of the pandemic virus to produce severe illness or death. This concept is only partially correct. First of all, it is important to remember that even if the hospitalization and mortality rates are not higher in a given pandemic than seen with seasonal influenza, the attack rates are two to four times higher and therefore the number of patients needing to be admitted to the hospital or dying will also be higher. Furthermore, pandemics often cause rapid peaks of illness which strain, and at times overwhelm, the capacity of the healthcare systems in many countries to care for those not only with influenza, but also other types of diseases.

Each pandemic has some unique features and these can impact the severity of the pandemic. In the 2009 pandemic, the risk of hospitalization and death was relatively low in otherwise healthy people including those

>65 years of age, but higher than expected in children, young and middle-aged adults with certain chronic diseases and dramatically greater in pregnant women, especially those women who also had asthma.[96] The lower risk of infection in people >65 of age was due to their low incidence of infection due to the substantial number of elderly people who had preexisting antibodies that neutralized the 2009 H1N1 virus. Those elderly people who did get infected were at high risk of complications (they had the second highest mortality rate/population which was only exceeded by 50–64-year-olds). Another important factor impacting the morbidity and mortality seen in the 2009 pandemic was that the incidence of some of the underlying risk factors, such as obesity, had increased substantially since the last pandemic in 1968. The net result was that while the overall mortality rate was similar to that seen with seasonal influenza, the absolute number of life years lost substantially increased in those with underlying medical conditions.

6.1.4 *Expanding Medical Surge Capacity*

Healthcare facilities typically maintain limited inventories of supplies on-site and depend on just-in-time restocking programs. Replenishment of critical inventories is therefore dependent upon an intact supply chain from manufacturing to transportation and receiving. During a pandemic, it is recognized that there will be an increased demand for both consumable (e.g., oseltamivir, masks) and durable (e.g., ventilators) resources. In addition to the pre-pandemic stockpiling of supplies and drugs, another very helpful program in the USA was that the federal government agreed to reimburse hospitals and physician practices for the cost of many of the pandemic-related supplies and drugs they purchased. This reimbursement policy allowed medical centers the flexibility to stockpile these items prior to the onset of the 2009 pandemic.

While the 2009 pandemic impacted many communities, each community experienced the pandemic as a local event and healthcare resources could not be easily redistributed as large numbers of people became ill over a short period of time. Many countries were forced to cancel routine appointments and elective procedures because of inadequate outpatient and emergency department capacity, shortages of inpatient beds particularly in the ICUs, and high numbers of HCWs who were out of work due to their own illness or to take care of an ill family member. In some countries insufficient numbers of intensive care beds and ventilators were available to treat all the patients requiring this level of care which further increased the number of deaths.

In the USA and other countries the number of persons seeking medical care during the second wave of the pandemic increased dramatically in many communities and overcrowding of outpatient and inpatient facilities occurred despite the planning and stockpiling that had previously occurred. A majority of those seeking care were managed appropriately by outpatient providers using a home-based approach. Appropriate management of outpatient pandemic influenza cases, including the early use of oseltamivir in those at high risk of complications, reduced the risk of progression to severe disease and thereby decreased the burden on healthcare providers and hospitals.

The surge plans created at medical centers helped deal with the increase in patients seeking medical care. Despite these plans, the capacity at many centers was stressed due to a marked increase in patients seeking care in the emergency department, increased incidence of absenteeism due to illness in HCWs or their family members and shortages of available inpatient beds particularly in the pediatric and adult ICUs. The increased number of patients with influenza also impacted the ability to provide care for patients with other types of medical and surgical conditions, particularly those needing elective procedures. Consideration of triage principles occurred in various medical centers to help decide which patients gained access to scarce medical resources (e.g., ECMO).

One way of accessing the overall effectiveness of the **Strategy** in mitigating the impact of the 2009 pandemic in the USA is to compare the estimated number of hospitalizations and deaths that occurred during the 2009 pandemic to some of the predictive models that were used to plan for a pandemic (Table 20). The number of infected patients, hospitalizations and deaths noted in Table 20 are based on an estimation methodology developed by the CDC that relies on a nationwide surveillance system

Table 20. The Estimated Actual Impact of the 2009 Pandemic Compared to What Was Predicted by Modeling Done by the CDC in 2005 and the President's Council of Advisors on Science and Technology (PCAST) in 2009*

Characteristic	CDC Pre-Pandemic Planning Modeling	PCAST Pre-Pandemic Planning Modeling	Estimated Actual Impact of the 2009 Pandemic[¶]
Illness	90 million (30%)	60–120 million	39–80 million (55 million)
Hospitalization	865,000	1–2 million	173,000 to 362,000 (246,000)
ICU care	128,750	150,000–300,000	10–30% of hospitalized cases[§]
Death	209,000	30,000–90,000	7,800–16,460 (11,160)

*The 2009 pandemic was considered to be of moderate severity. The 2005 CDC modeling for a moderate pandemic was based on the 1957 and 1968 pandemic which were also considered moderate. The PCAST modeling was based on the 1968 pandemic.

[¶]The data noted for the 2009 pandemic are preliminary estimates from the start of the pandemic in April until December 12, 2009. The numbers in parentheses are the mid-range values (www.cdc.gov/h1n1flu/estimates_2009_h1n1.htm).[69]

[§]The estimated percentage of hospitalized patients infected with the 2009 H1N1 virus that needed ICU care. The CDC has not yet reported an estimate of the actual number of ICU cases.

and statistical modeling.[69] Like other pandemics, the 2009 pandemic had its own unique features (e.g., the majority of deaths were due to 2009 H1N1 viral pneumonia rather than secondary bacterial infections, the elderly were relatively less susceptible to the 2009 H1N1 virus infection and therefore fewer deaths occurred in this group than anticipated, etc.) that directly impacted the hospitalization and mortality rates independent of any impact of the **Strategy**. However, there is substantial evidence that some of the planning steps did have an impact on the number of hospitalizations and deaths (e.g., the ready availability of oseltamivir due to the existing stockpiles, the availability of pandemic vaccine for some high-priority groups during the second wave, etc.).

6.2 The Need to Review Pandemic Planning from a Global Perspective

Influenza pandemics are a global disease and require each country to have their own plans that then need to become part of a well-thought-out coordinated worldwide strategy if we are to further mitigate the impact of the next pandemic. In January 2010, the WHO Executive Board requested a proposal from the WHO Director-General on how to assess the international response to the 2009 pandemic and approved her suggestion to convene the International Health Regulations Review Committee to review the 2009 pandemic response (http://www.who.int/csr/disease/swineflu/ frequently_asked_questions/review_committee/en/index.html). The International Health Regulations is an international legal agreement that is binding on 194 countries across the globe, including all of the WHO Member States. The basic purpose of the International Health Regulations is to help the international community prevent and respond to acute public health risks that have the potential to cross borders and threaten people worldwide. In arranging the 2009 pandemic review, the WHO aimed to facilitate a process that was independent, credible and transparent and offered a critical assessment of how the WHO and the international community responded to the pandemic.

The assessment of the global response to the 2009 began in April 2010 and is being conducted by the International Health Regulations Review Committee that is composed of experts from around the world who have a broad mix of scientific expertise and practical experience in public health. The Review Committee is chaired by Professor Harvey V. Fineberg, President of the Institute of Medicine, Washington DC, and has 28 other members — the list of members can be found at http://www.who.int/ihr/r_c_members/en/index.html.

The purpose of this review was to aid the management of future public health emergencies of international concern. Specifically the Review Committee was asked to: 1) assess the functioning of the International Health Regulations (2005) in relation to the current pandemic (H1N1) (2009) and other public health events, 2) to review the scope, appropriateness, effectiveness and responsiveness of global actions as well as the role of the WHO Secretariat in supporting pandemic preparedness, alert and response in relation to the pandemic, and 3) based on the above, to identify and review the major lessons learnt from the global response to the current pandemic and to recommend actions to be taken by Member States and the

Director-General to strengthen the preparedness and response to potential future influenza pandemics and other public health emergencies. The tentative schedule for the Committee's work includes a number of in-person meetings, teleconferences and electronic exchanges with a final report to be presented to the Sixty-fourth World Health Assembly in May 2011. Documents from various meetings and teleconferences will be posted on the website (http://www.who.int/ihr/review_committee/en/index.html).

There are many lessons to be learned from the 2009 pandemic that will enable us to better plan for the next pandemic. Analysis of what occurred will not stop with the final report of the International Health Regulations Review Committee or other ongoing reviews, but rather will be studied by many public health officials and researchers for many years. While no one can predict with certainty when the next pandemic will occur, one thing is clear: there will be other pandemics in the 21st century! The next pandemic will have important similarities and differences from the 2009 pandemic, but the more we learn about past pandemics the better we can prepare for future ones.

References

93. Sustaining global surveillance and response to emerging zoonotic diseases. (2009) Institute of Medicine, September, 1–6 [www.iom.edu/zoonotic diseases].
94. Bristol N. (2009) US targets disease prevention in health reforms. *Lancet* **374**: 1957–1958.
95. Ready or not? Protecting the public's health from disease, disasters, and bioterrorism. (2009) Trust for America's Health, December [http://healthyamericans.org/reports/bioterror09].
96. Siston AM, Rasmussen SA, Honein MA *et al.*; Pandemic H1N1 Influenza in Pregnancy Working Group. (2010) Pandemic 2009 influenza A(H1N1) virus illness among pregnant women in the United States. *JAMA* **303**: 1517–1525.

Chapter 7

Mitigating the Impact of the Next Pandemic

"Prediction is very difficult, especially if it's about the future."

Niels Bohr

7.1 Research Studies and Policy Changes Needed to Better Deal with the Next Pandemic

The final chapter in this book discusses new knowledge and policy changes that should be considered to achieve the goal of substantially mitigating the impact of the next pandemic. The research questions and policy issues noted in this chapter are just some of those that if answered would help better predict when the next influenza pandemic will occur and allow the development of a global strategy to mitigate its impact. Many of the questions included in specific sections of this chapter are pertinent to other sections (e.g., both host and viral factors can interact to impact the transmissibility and severity of influenza disease). Some of the studies that would provide answers to these questions are noted in the bulleted parts in this chapter. The results of these studies and policies will also help in the future to better deal with seasonal influenza and other emerging infections.

7.1.1 *Research Questions Pertaining to Influenza Viruses*

> A KEY POINT: Our knowledge about influenza viruses has come a long way and yet there is still a great deal that needs to be determined. For example, the ability to sequence the genome of these viruses has been available for over two decades, but the genetic determinants that control the ability of the virus to transmit easily between people, one of the necessary characteristics for an influenza virus to cause a pandemic, still needs to be determined.

1) What are the genetic components of the virus that determine the impact of the virus on the human population?

The extent and severity of disease caused by influenza viruses vary substantially both with seasonal and pandemic influenza. While some of this variability relates to the human host, it is clear that genetic properties of the virus also play a major role. Some of the studies that are needed include those determining:

• Factors that control the genetic exchange of material between human and animal influenza viruses.
• Why, at least for the past century, widespread global human disease has been limited to infections with H1N1, H2N2 and H3N2 strains when there are 16 HA and 9 NA proteins which equates to 144 possible combinations of influenza A viruses that could potentially cause widespread disease in humans.
• Genetic determinants in influenza viruses that impact the transmissibility and virulence of the virus.

2) What are the major environmental factors that result in the virus causing seasonal disease in temperate countries and outbreaks throughout the year in tropical countries?

Influenza viruses cause disease mainly in the winter months in temperate countries in the Northern and Southern Hemispheres. In contrast, in tropical countries outbreaks of disease occur year-round. While there is evidence indicating that low humidity favors the viability of the virus, this factor alone does not fully explain this variance in disease pattern. Furthermore, as the 2009 pandemic has shown, large outbreaks of disease can occur in temperate countries during the summer months. Needed studies include those determining:

- Other environmental factors that influence when outbreaks of influenza disease will occur.
- Environmental conditions that affect the genetic mutations that occur in influenza viruses, including the ability of the virus to recombine genetic material from various species.
- The role of the environment in allowing influenza viruses to predominate over many of these other types of respiratory viruses during influenza virus season.
- How global warming might alter the way influenza viruses spread across the globe.

3) What components of the virus are important in causing severe complications?

Each year the most common complication of influenza that leads to hospitalization and death is secondary bacterial infections. However, the 2009 pandemic was an exception to this rule and most of the patients admitted to the ICUs, including those who died, appeared to have a primary viral pneumonia often in association with ARDS. A recently published study using a ferret animal model suggested that intratracheal inoculation with the 2009 H1N1 virus caused more widespread disease throughout the respiratory tract of these animals than a 2007 seasonal H1N1 virus which replicated mainly in the bronchi.[97] Of interest was the finding that the H5N1 virus, which also causes severe viral pneumonitis, resulted in the most severe pulmonary disease. Further studies are needed to examine the importance of these findings in humans and other studies are needed to examine:

- Other viral factors that predispose patients to primary viral versus secondary bacterial pneumonia.

7.1.2 *Research Questions Pertaining to Clinical Disease*

> A KEY POINT: A few studies in the literature suggest that some otherwise healthy people in certain families are genetically predisposed to more severe disease, but other studies come to the opposite conclusion. If a genetic susceptibility exists and can be defined then these high-risk families can be prioritized for prevention and early intervention modalities.

Those who suffer serious morbidity and mortality due to seasonal and pandemic influenza usually are those with chronic underlying disease, particularly those who are elderly. However, each year a substantial percentage of those who are hospitalized or die due to influenza have no identifiable underlying condition. A better understanding of what other currently unidentified risk factors predispose otherwise healthy patients to severe disease due to influenza and the pathogenesis of severe disease in those with risk factors would help identify those who should be targeted for prevention and help improve the treatment of those who develop severe disease.

1) What, if any, are the host genetic factors that determine why most people infected with influenza viruses remain asymptomatic or develop only mild disease while others develop severe disease?

While underlying risk factors are an important reason why people develop severe disease due to seasonal and pandemic influenza viruses, a substantial minority of the severe cases have no underlying risk factors. Currently, there is conflicting evidence about whether there is a genetic susceptibility that explains why some otherwise healthy people develop severe influenza. A retrospective study involving the 1918 pandemic examined this question.[98] For over three centuries the entire population of Iceland has been closely tracked using a de-CODE genealogic database. The investigators in this study examined the relative importance of risk of exposure to an influenza virus-infected person(s) versus genetic susceptibility in the development of severe disease. They concluded that most, if not all, of the increased risk to severe disease could be explained by the risk of exposure.

In contrast, another retrospective study used the Utah Population Database, a genealogic resource of people who originally settled in Utah and their descendants, to address this question.[99] These investigators looked at death certificates in Utah over a 100-year period and found an increased risk of death due to influenza not only in first-degree relatives, but also in second- and third-degree relatives. They concluded that the increased risk in more distant relatives who did not have exposure to each other at the time of their illness strongly supported the concept that genetic risk factors were an important cause of death due to influenza.

Dr. Francis Collins, the current director of the NIH and formerly the head of the National Human Genome Research Institute where he had a major role in leading the effort to sequence the human genome, has predicted that during the next decade the genetic makeup of each individual will become part of their medical background information. Achieving this goal would offer a unique opportunity to determine the true extent to which genetic susceptibilities determine an individual's risk of developing severe influenza. High risk individuals could be prioritized for prevention of disease using influenza vaccines or antiviral prophylaxis in addition to early treatment if they develop disease. Potential studies include examining if there are host genetic determinants that:

- Increase or decrease the risk of someone developing severe disease.
- Enable an infected individual to remain asymptomatic.
- Are specific for various types of complications (e.g., viral pneumonia, secondary bacterial pneumonia, encephalopathy, etc.).

2) What other risk factors increase the risk of hospitalization or death in those with no currently identifiable underlying risk factors?

During the 2009 pandemic, obesity was identified as a new possible risk factor for the development of severe influenza disease. There are likely a number of other risk factors that lead to severe disease that have not yet been identified. For example, a recent study done during the 2009 pandemic suggested that immunoglobulin G2 subclass deficiency may be a previously unidentified risk factor for severe disease.[100] Some of these patients with immunoglobulin G2 deficiency had other known risk factors (e.g., pregnancy), but others had no known risk factors. Additional studies are needed to:

- Identify additional risk factors in apparently healthy individuals who develop severe disease.
- Determine if the coexistence of two or more risk factors in a given patient increases their risk, and if so, which risk factors and by how much.

3) What specific factors increase the risk of hospitalization or death in those with certain underlying chronic diseases?

There are multiple chronic diseases that increase the risk of developing severe complications from seasonal and pandemic influenza. Understanding the specific factors that contribute to this risk for each of the chronic diseases is important for finding ways to prevent this from happening. Needed studies include those determining if there are:

- Only a few common pathways by which these chronic diseases lead to severe disease or if most chronic diseases have their own specific pathway.
- Genetic determinants for each of these chronic diseases that increase the risk for those who develop severe disease.

4) What is the pathogenesis of the severe disease that occurs at a markedly increased rate in pregnant women infected with influenza virus?

The risk of hospitalization for healthy pregnant women infected with a seasonal influenza virus is ∼3 times higher than that for healthy non-pregnant women of similar age. In pandemics, the risk of hospitalization and death is even greater, and in the 2009 pandemic, the reported risk was as much as 10 times higher. The risk of severe disease increases over each trimester and remains increased for up to a month postpartum. Studies to elucidate the reasons why the risk for severe disease is so high in pregnant women include determining:

- The role that the immunologic changes that occur in pregnant women, enabling them to not reject their fetus, have in increasing the risk of pregnant women developing severe disease due to influenza virus.
- If the impact of decreased lung compliance due to the growing fetus is the main reason for the increased risk of severe disease.
- Why the risk for severe disease is so much greater for influenza than other respiratory viruses.

7.1.3 *Research Questions and Policy Issues Pertaining to Prevention and Treatment of Influenza*

> A KEY POINT: The Holy Grail for prevention of influenza would be the development of a safe vaccine that is efficacious against all influenza virus strains and does not need to be given annually. Various groups have been working on this idea for years; however, such a vaccine is likely years away.

There are a number of problems with the current influenza vaccine program, including how the effectiveness of the current vaccine varies based on how well the strains in the vaccine match those that are circulating in the populations, the vaccine has to be given on a yearly basis, vaccine production problems occur frequently, and the majority of those who are recommended to get the vaccine do not do so. In addition to improving our ability to prevent infection, new modalities are needed to more effectively treat some of the complications that currently cause hospitalization and death. Some of the questions that need to be addressed in order to improve the ability to prevent and treat influenza include:

1) What can be done to improve the reliability and speed of the current manufacturing process used to make influenza vaccines?

The most common reason why the seasonal trivalent influenza vaccine is delayed during production is due to one or more of the viral strains contained in the vaccine not growing well in eggs. During the first and second waves of the 2009 pandemic, the amount of vaccine produced fell far short of what was predicted or needed. The anticipated worldwide production capacity for pandemic vaccine had been markedly revised downward from an annual production of 4.5 billion doses predicted in June 2009 to a revised estimate in January 2010 of 1,296,000,000 doses (~29% of what had been predicted) due in large part to lower than expected yields of the HA protein and continuing manufacturing issues.

As the second wave was receding in November 2009, USA Health and Human Services Secretary Kathleen Sebelius noted that the shortage of H1N1 vaccine indicated that the USA depended on antiquated technology. She felt that the government's response to the pandemic was adequate, as the process of identifying the virus, producing and distributing diagnostic tests, and launching an immunization campaign was undertaken as quickly as possible. However, Secretary Sebelius stated that, "We were fighting the 2009 H1N1 flu with vaccine technology from the 1950s. We could race to begin vaccine production, but there was nothing we could do if vaccine grew slowly in eggs. We could make deals with foreign vaccine producers ahead of time, but we still wouldn't have as much control over the vaccine production and distribution as if they were based in the USA."

A great deal has been learned over the past several decades about critical factors that can impact the growth of the virus and yet this problem continues to occur. One step that is clearly needed is to increase the number of manufacturers in developing countries. Additionally, further research studies are needed to:

- Develop procedures that allow consistent and predictable growth of seasonal and pandemic vaccine virus strains.
- Examine the critical factors that determine how well influenza viruses grow in eggs and in cell cultures.
- Further develop the capacity to make very large quantities of influenza vaccine using newer methods (e.g., recombinant antigen technology, DNA-based vaccines, viral vectors, etc.).

- Develop methods to streamline the manufacturing steps involved in producing very large quantities of vaccine doses once the raw material that makes up the vaccine is ready to be packaged.

2) Are there viral component(s) that are common to all influenza viruses and that can elicit long-lasting protection against a wide variety of influenza A and B strains?

Studies are needed to:

- Produce vaccines viral components that are internal or external to the viral envelope that elicit a broadly protective immune response to influenza A and B strains.
- Further develop additives (e.g., adjuvants) and find different routes of immunization (e.g., intradermal) to induce a more robust and prolonged immune response particularly in young children and the elderly.

3) Can more effective communication methods be developed to educate the public about vaccines, including complex issues such as risk versus benefit and association versus causation?

The use of vaccines, for centuries, starting with the smallpox vaccine, has generated controversy. The concern by some members of the public about the safety of vaccines recommended for their children or themselves appears to have become more prevalent during the last couple of decades. In part this concern is due to the decreasing incidence of vaccine-preventable diseases (e.g., polio, measles, etc.) and the ready availability of information, accurate and inaccurate, that can be obtained via the internet. While media coverage makes it seem like many more people are refusing vaccines, the actual data suggests that there is still strong support for vaccines, but there is a minority of the population who feel differently and they tend to congregate in certain communities.

A study by Gust *et al.*[101] described five different groups of parents that included those who are immunization advocates (33%), go along with others (26%), are health advocates (25%), fence-sitters (13%) and worriers (3%). We need to better understand the belief systems and concerns of individuals who are refusing vaccinations and find ways to help the public understand the various scientific methods and evidence that go into recommendations for the use of vaccines. For the public to truly understand the reason why public health authorities recommend the use of both seasonal and pandemic influenza vaccines, people need to have a better understanding of two complex topics: 1) the risk versus benefit of a vaccine for an individual/family and for the population as a whole and 2) what side effects are actually caused by the vaccine rather than those simply associated with receipt of the vaccine. These are difficult enough subjects for scientists to grapple with, no less the general public.

The concern about whether influenza vaccine causes GBS highlights some of the issues related to these two topics. Even if one believes that the 2009 H1N1 vaccine could cause GBS at a rate similar to that associated with the 1976 swine influenza vaccine ($\sim$1 case per 100,000 people vaccinated), the reduction of morbidity and mortality derived from receiving the vaccine outweighs this risk on a population basis. However, an otherwise healthy individual might reasonably assess the risk of getting GBS due to the vaccine as being greater than that of developing severe disease from the 2009 H1N1 virus.

The decision to recommend the pandemic vaccine to the entire USA population clearly meant that vaccination of some individuals would be associated with the occurrence of GBS since a certain number of individuals would develop GBS even if the vaccine was not given. Thus, for someone who develops GBS within a 2–6-week time frame of receipt of the vaccine, their belief that the vaccine is causally, rather than just temporally, related to the onset of GBS is plausible since this is within a time frame that the vaccine could have induced antibodies that could cause such an autoimmune disease. To address this possibility, the WHO and CDC worked with various countries to develop a pandemic vaccine safety monitoring system that included an intense surveillance system for GBS. This system was initiated prior to the availability of the vaccine as well as during the time the vaccine was being given to the public. These data will allow a much better determination of whether these two events (i.e., receipt of the vaccine and occurrence of GBS) are causally related, and if so, how frequently GBS is caused by the vaccine rather than the virus itself or some other etiologic agent.

To date, only a minority of those recommended to get the seasonal and pandemic influenza vaccines actually do so. Studies are needed to examine how to most effectively:

- Educate the public on the topics of risk versus benefit and temporal association versus causation.
- Communicate with the public about who should be vaccinated and why.

4) How can "herd protection" most effectively be achieved using influenza vaccine?

A number of studies suggest, but do not conclusively prove, that a vaccination program that concentrates on immunizing school-age children can reduce the burden of influenza disease in the rest of the population (i.e., result in herd protection). The Japanese used to routinely immunize all school-age children and this was associated with a decreased incidence of disease in the elderly.[102] A more recent study done in the Hutterite communities in Canada provided further evidence that immunizing children and adolescents provides protection to unimmunized residents in the same communities.[103] Therefore, these studies were done during epidemic years and to date evidence is lacking that demonstrates this approach would be effective in a pandemic where often the attack rate is high and vaccine is in short supply. To demonstrate that initially focusing the use of vaccine on school-age children is a strategy that helps maximize the impact of the vaccine for the whole community, further studies are needed to:

- Clearly demonstrate that herd protection can be achieved with such a strategy that focuses on immunizing school-age children in the setting of seasonal influenza and determining what percentage of school-age children need to be vaccinated to achieve herd protection.

- Develop better models, using the information from the above studies, to predict the impact of such a strategy in the setting of mild, moderate and severe pandemics.

5) How can influenza viral pneumonia and the accompanying ARDS be treated more effectively?

One of the unique aspects of the 2009 pandemic when compared to both seasonal influenza and past pandemics is that most deaths appeared to be due to primary viral pneumonia and ARDS rather than secondary bacterial pneumonia. For the H5N1 virus, the development of ARDS in patients appeared to be due, at least in part, to a "cytokine storm" occurring as part of the immunologic response to the H5N1 virus. Clinicians have attempted to treat the virus-induced ARDS by using drugs that decrease the release of these cytokines. However, a recent study suggests that the 2009 pandemic virus does not induce a potent cytokine response.[104] Further basic, translational and well-controlled multi-center clinical studies are needed to:

- Develop additional antiviral agents that work against influenza virus via mechanisms that are different from those of the currently available drugs.
- Determine the pathogenesis of the influenza virus-induced ARDS and how to better treat it.

6) What policy changes are needed to help deal with surge capacity issues that impact that quality of care during a pandemic?

An increased number of HCWs were out of work during the 2009 pandemic. While much of the increase in absenteeism was due to the HCWs themselves being ill, some HCWs stayed home to care for a family member infected with the 2009 H1N1 virus. High HCW absenteeism can impact the quality of care patients receive. This problem raises the question of whether the families of HCWs should also be given high priority for pandemic vaccine when there is insufficient supply to vaccinate everyone. In 2005, when the initial pandemic vaccine prioritization scheme was being developed by the USA government, this issue was raised, but the ethicists who participated in the meeting felt that giving high priority for vaccine to families of HCWs could not be ethically justified. A reassessment of the benefits and costs of including family members of HCWs as high priority is needed. If the benefits to patient care are substantial then the ethical considerations regarding immunizing the families of HCWs would need to be reconsidered in light of the number of people who suffer adverse events due to the decreased quality of care.

7.1.4 *Research Questions and Policy Issues Pertaining to Resolving Resource Equity Issues Between Developed and Developing Countries*

> A KEY POINT: A great deal of epidemiologic research has been done in the area of influenza, but there is still very little known about the extent to which the morbidity and mortality due to influenza is greater in developing countries than in developed countries and the most important factors contributing to this problem. While the answers to these questions would not fix the problem of inequitable distribution of vaccines, drugs and supplies used to prevent and treat influenza, they could heighten the political pressure to deal with the medical, social and ethical problems that cause these inequities.

1) What are the major underlying factors that cause severe morbidity and mortality due to influenza in developing countries?

Given the fact that many developing countries have poorly functioning health systems, a relatively young demographic profile, widespread prevalence of co-morbidities and chronic conditions such as malnutrition, HIV/AIDS and tuberculosis, the impact of seasonal and pandemic influenza will likely have a larger impact on developing countries compared to developed ones. For example, the increased risk of death among pregnant women in South Africa infected with the 2009 H1N1 virus was reported to be greater in pregnant women infected with HIV versus those without HIV.[105] The lack of certainty about the impact of influenza on these countries is due to the paucity of epidemiologic and interventional studies that have examined this issue. These types of studies are critical in order to provide information on the most effective ways to decrease the impact of influenza in these countries and how to best utilize available resources to do so.

2) What criteria should be used to decide how scarce resources are utilized during a pandemic?

Many medical centers in both developed and developing countries ran out or came perilously close to not having enough essential resources that were needed to care for those who were hospitalized with disease due to the 2009 H1N1 virus. In developed countries, the problem was most acute for those who were severely ill and needed ICU care. Even in those medical centers where the problem was not severe enough to make triage of these resources necessary during the first and second waves, many centers began to develop a protocol to determine how they would deal with this issue if it did occur. Such a dire situation calls for policies that preemptively determine who should receive scarce resources (e.g., ICU beds, ventilators, etc.). The protocol is intended to guide decisions about access to intensive care for all patients who need these resources, not just influenza virus-infected patients. The steps that would be taken would be a major departure from normal practice, and implemented only in the event that the number of patients requiring these resources exceeds what is available. Modeling of these protocols is needed and the best ones need to be considered for widespread distribution. These policies could also be helpful in severe epidemic influenza seasons and in certain other widespread emergencies.

3) What is the appropriate role for adjuvanted vaccines in helping to reduce the inequitable distribution of vaccines between developed and developing countries?

The manufacturing capacity for influenza vaccines is large globally, yet there was still not enough vaccine available to immunize the world's population during the first and second waves of the 2009 pandemic. The great majority of production capacity for the pandemic vaccine had already been reserved by industrialized countries. Studies indicated that the amount of virus material in at least some of the pandemic vaccine formulations that contained adjuvants could be decreased substantially and allow ~4 times as many people to be immunized against the H1N1 virus when compared to unadjuvanted vaccines.

Various considerations went into the decision on whether to use adjuvanted 2009 H1N1 virus vaccines. Less vaccine than expected was produced due to manufacturing problems. This production problem further decreased the amount of vaccine that developing countries would initially receive and the use of adjuvanted vaccines helped overcome this problem. Another potential advantage associated with the use of adjuvanted vaccines is that it often induces broader protection against influenza viruses and this is particularly helpful when the circulating and vaccine strains are not well matched. However, the 2009 H1N1 virus has not undergone substantial genetic changes and therefore the vaccine strain was well matched to the circulating 2009 H1N1 virus.

Potential disadvantages of using adjuvanted vaccines include that the safety of different adjuvants used by various manufacturers had not been previously fully demonstrated for influenza vaccines and this lack of information raised public fears about vaccine safety. In the USA, adjuvanted vaccines had not been previously approved by the Food and Drug Administration and therefore their use would have to occur under an Emergency Use Authorization. Furthermore, preliminary data from studies using unadjuvanted vaccines suggested that even without an adjuvant, a single injection, rather than the previously predicted two doses, of unadjuvanted pandemic vaccines conferred protection in those > 10 years of age. To a certain extent, these studies decreased the pressure on the USA government to use adjuvanted vaccines since by November 2009 the USA determined it had contracts for more vaccine doses then it would likely need and could donate some of its vaccine supply to the WHO.

With developing countries facing severe shortages of the pandemic vaccine, the WHO recommended the use of adjuvants to increase the number of people who could be vaccinated. While many developed nations decided to use adjuvanted vaccines, the USA government decided to only use unadjuvanted vaccines. The use of adjuvanted vaccines helped increase the global supply of vaccine during the 2009 pandemic and could increase the number of vaccine doses even more if all countries would use adjuvanted vaccine, going forward, to prevent both seasonal and pandemic influenza.

4) What other steps can be taken to ensure that developing countries have equitable access to resources to prevent and treat influenza?

Global supplies of the two most important interventional items — vaccines and antiviral medications — are constrained, in part due to their cost. More than 1 billion vaccine doses had been ordered from the various vaccine companies, and nearly all the "customers" were the governments of the 15 wealthiest nations in the world. The sale of the H1N1 vaccine to these countries was a very profitable endeavor for many vaccine manufacturers. For example, by August 2009, GlaxoSmithKline (GSK) had received a total order of 291 million doses of pandemic vaccine, and this was estimated to make the company a $3 billion profit.[106] Developed countries and for-profit vaccine manufacturers have a responsibility to help ensure that vaccines are distributed fairly to all countries. By the time of the SAGE meeting in April 2010, five major influenza vaccine manufacturers (GSK, Sanofi-Aventis, Novartis, MedImmune and CSL) had agreed to donate millions of doses of the pandemic vaccine to the WHO for use in developing countries. In addition, 12 developed countries (Australia, Brazil, France, Germany, Italy, Japan, New Zealand, Norway, Switzerland, Thailand, the United Kingdom and the USA) announced that they would donate up to 10% of their 2009 pandemic vaccine supply to the WHO for use in low-income countries. In total these donations were estimated to allow the WHO to allocate ~190 million doses to developing countries.

The issue of pharmaceutical company profits came to a head towards the end of 2009, when Wolfgang Wodarg, Chairman of the Health Committee of the Parliamentary Assembly of the Council of Europe, accused the WHO of being improperly influenced by the pharmaceutical industry. The press gave this story wide coverage and some of the articles went as far as calling the 2009 pandemic "fake", suggesting that the 2009 pandemic was contrived to increase profits in the pharmaceutical industry.[107] These allegations ignored many of the factual events that led to the WHO declaring the pandemic, including the large number of hospitalizations and deaths that were occurring in Mexico at the onset of the pandemic, the rapid transmission of a unique recombinant influenza virus globally, and the severity of disease in pregnant women and those with underlying chronic health conditions. The accusation that some members of SAGE and other WHO advisory groups had conflicts of interest that were not properly managed by the WHO was also unfounded. The WHO is a specialized agency of the United Nations with 193 member countries and must collaborate with many organizations, including industry, to fulfill its mission of improving the health of the world's population. The conflict-of-interest vetting process for each WHO advisory group member is transparent, thorough and well-managed.[108]

To reduce the adverse effects of pandemic influenza in developing countries, the Bill & Melinda Gates Foundation continued to work with governments in various developed countries, companies and other organizations to help developing countries gain access to the 2009 pandemic influenza vaccines in a timely fashion. The use of these vaccines was seen as the most effective way to mitigate the impact of the 2009 pandemic. As a result of these discussions, the Gates Foundation proposed several principles for global allocation of pandemic vaccines (http://www.gatesfoundation.org/topics/Pages/pneumonia-flu.aspx). The hope was that these principles would stimulate discussion of potential actions to be taken by these groups to ensure equitable access to vaccines during the 2009 and subsequent pandemics. The adherence to these below noted recommendations and the impact that they have needs to be assessed.

- The global community should take steps to protect all populations, including those without resources to protect themselves.

- Vaccination should be considered in the context of comprehensive pandemic preparedness and response efforts in all nations.
- Developed countries and vaccine manufacturers should urgently agree upon a mechanism to ensure access to vaccines by developing countries.
- Influenza vaccine manufacturers should identify strategies such as tiered pricing and/or donations to make pandemic vaccines more accessible to developing nations.
- Pandemic vaccines allocated to developing nations should become available in the same time frame as vaccines for developed nations.
- The global community should obtain data to help establish a consensus on the safety and efficacy of adjuvants, and efforts should be made to ensure the fullest use of this and other dose-sparing strategies.
- All countries obtaining pandemic vaccines should ensure that mechanisms are in place to provide this vaccine to their populations, to ensure this scarce resource is not wasted, and donors should be prepared to provide resources and technical assistance to help countries bolster these mechanisms.
- The WHO is uniquely positioned to lead the global response to a pandemic virus and should support governments and industry in their efforts to implement these principles.

Another strategy involves technical and financial support from developed countries and other entities to help developing countries further develop their own vaccine manufacturing capacity. The WHO is managing an ambitious technology project for influenza vaccine production involving 11 manufacturers in developing countries. Some countries, such as China, Korea and Romania, have already manufactured influenza vaccines and were able to manufacture pandemic vaccines for their own population. Two manufacturers in India and Thailand conducted clinical trials of pandemic vaccines in late 2009 to early 2010. While in the foreseeable future it is unlikely that every country will be able to develop its own internal capacity to make vaccines, it is possible that various developing countries can create agreements that would be mutually beneficial. For example, a country that decides to develop the capacity to make influenza vaccines could enter into an agreement with other countries to sell them seasonal vaccines on an annual basis and pandemic vaccines when needed. The annual sale of influenza vaccines in larger quantities then needed just for the population of the country manufacturing the vaccine would help make the business venture more viable and also help meet the needs of the other countries that are part of the agreement.

Many developed countries had purchased or contracted for large quantities of oseltamivir (and to a lesser extent, zanamivir) and personal protective equipment (e.g., various types of masks) and these sales resulted in large profits for the manufacturers. Some of the developed countries and manufacturers did donate or sell these products at a reduced price, but very substantial inequities in the distribution of these items remained. Similar mechanisms to those proposed above for equitable distribution of vaccines need to be developed for antiviral agents and other supplies.

7.2 Some Final Thoughts

> A KEY POINT: The end of a pandemic really marks the beginning of the next pandemic. The virus is a chameleon and a warrior worthy of our continuous and full attention. Anything less will leave us in great peril.

The Director General of the WHO on August 10, 2010 announced that the 2009 H1N1 pandemic had ended and that we were now in the post-pandemic period. Soon thereafter, scientists at the USA National Institute of Health estimated that about 183 million Americans (~59% of the total USA population) had some immunity to the 2009 H1N1 virus due to pre-existing immunity prior to the pandemic, infection by the 2009 H1N1 virus or receipt of the vaccine (reference 109). The percentage of the world's population that now have some immunity to the 2009 H1N1 virus remains to be determined as does the impact of this virus going forward.

The impact of the 2009 pandemic was less severe than many had predicted, but not as mild as others have suggested. In part this was due to the pre-pandemic planning that had occurred. Many of those who now criticize various public health and government leaders for spending too much money on pandemic planning would be the same people who disparaging these groups for not doing enough if the pandemic had been more severe.

Influenza viruses undergo frequent changes and in a very real sense can be considered a continuously emerging infection. Much of what we learn about influenza is transferable to other emerging infections and a great deal of the infrastructure that is needed to deal with influenza can be synergistically used to identify and combat other emerging infections, including those that might be created for biological warfare. Without planning there will be no prevention and substantially less cure.

References

97. van den Brand JM, Stittelaar KJ, van Amerongen G *et al.* (2010) Severity of pneumonia due to new H1N1 influenza virus in ferrets is intermediate between that due to seasonal H1N1 virus and highly pathogenic avian influenza H5N1 virus. *J Infect Dis* **201**: 993–999.

98. Dowell SF, Bresee JS. (2008) Pandemic lessons from Iceland. *Proc Natl Acad Sci United States* **105**: 1109–1110.

99. Albright FS, Orlando P, Pavia AT *et al.* (2008) Evidence for a heritable predisposition to death due to influenza. *J Infect Dis* **197**: 1–3.

100. Gordon CL, Johnson PD, Permezel M *et al.* (2010) Association between severe pandemic 2009 influenza A (H1N1) virus infection and immunoglobulin G(2) subclass deficiency. *Clin Infect Dis* **50**: 672–678.

101. Gust DA, Brown C, Sheedy K *et al.* (2005) Immunization attitudes and beliefs among parents: Beyond a dichotomous perspective. *Am J Health Behav* **29**(1): 81–92.

102. Reichert TA, Sugaya N, Fedson DS *et al.* (2001) The Japanese experience with vaccinating school children against influenza. *N Engl J Med* **344**: 889–896.

103. Loeb M, Russell ML, Moss L *et al.* (2010) Effect of influenza vaccination of children on infection rates in Hutterite communities: A randomized trial. *JAMA* **303**: 943–950.

104. Woo PC, Tung ET, Chan KH *et al.* (2010) Cytokine profiles induced by the novel swine-origin influenza A/H1N1 virus: Implications for treatment strategies. *J Infect Dis* **201**: 346–353.

105. Archer B, Cohen C, Naidoo D *et al.* (2009) Interim report on pandemic H1N1 influenza virus infections in South Africa, April to October 2009: Epidemiology and factors associated with fatal cases. *Euro Surveill* **14**: pii19639.

106. Published letter to Council on Foreign Relations, White House H1N1 Report, August 27, 2009.

107. Statement of the World Health Organization on allegations of conflict of interest and 'fake' pandemic, January 22, 2010 [http://www.who.int/media-centre/news/statements/2010/h1n1_pandemic_20100122/en/index.html].

108. Statement by Dr. Keiji Fukuda on behalf of WHO at the Council of Europe hearing on pandemic (H1N1) 2009, January 26, 2010 [http://www.who.int/csr/disease/swineflu/coe_hearing/en/index.html].

109. Morens DM, Taubenburger JK, Fauci AS. (2001) The 2009 H1N1 pandemic influenza virus: What next? mBio Doi:10.1128/mBio.00211-10.

Acknowledgments

A number of people have generously given of their time to review this book and make helpful suggestions. These include Dr. Chris Ohl, Associate Professor of Medicine, Section on Infectious Diseases at Wake Forest University Baptist Medical Center; Dr. Philippe Duclos, Senior Health Adviser/SAGE Executive Secretary, Immunization Policy (ICP), Immunization, Vaccines and Biologicals (IVB); Dr. Larry Givner, Professor of Pediatrics, Section of Infectious Diseases at Wake Forest University Baptist Medical Center; Dr. Marie-Paule Kieny, Director, Initiatives for Vaccine Research (IVR), Immunizations, Vaccines and Biologicals (IVB); Dr. Cynthia Lees, Assistant Professor of Pathology, Section on Comparative Medicine at Wake Forest University Baptist Medical Center; Dr. Stephen Reed, Director of the CDC Influenza Coordination Unit; Professor David M. Salisbury, Director of Immunisation, United Kingdom Department of Health; and Dr. Robert Sherertz, Associate Professor of Medicine, Section on Infectious Diseases at Wake Forest University Baptist Medical Center.

Index

www.ingramcontent.com/pod-product-compliance
Lightning Source LLC
Chambersburg PA
CBHW050627190326
41458CB00008B/2164